Helping Your Breech Baby Turn

A Comprehensive Guide for Expectant Mothers with Natural Practices and Expert Tips to Safely Turn Your Baby

Mary Shaw

Contents

Table of Contents

INTRODUCTION

The act of bringing a new life into the world is a profound and life-altering process that is accompanied by feelings of anticipation, excitement, and frequently a good deal of fear. The position of the baby in the womb is a key aspect that can impact the course of pregnancy and birth. This is just one of the many problems that pregnant parents may have to deal with.

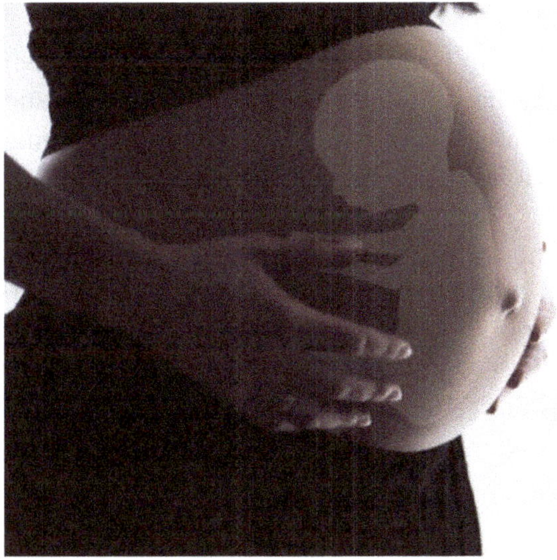

A scenario in which the baby is positioned with their buttocks or feet first, rather than the preferred head-first position, is referred to as breech presentation. "Helping Your Breech Baby Turn" is a comprehensive guide that aims to provide parents and caregivers with the knowledge and tools necessary to understand and address breech presentation.

Understanding Breech Position

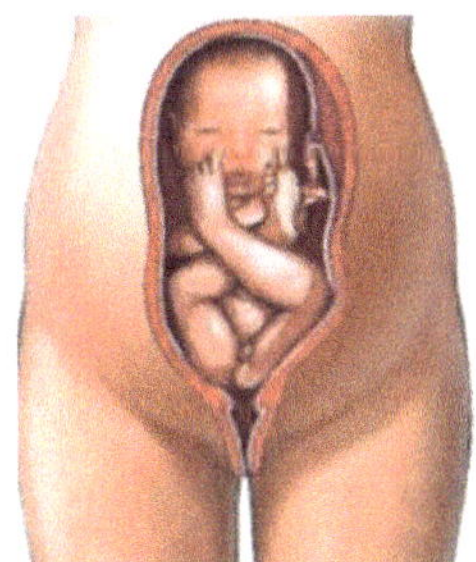
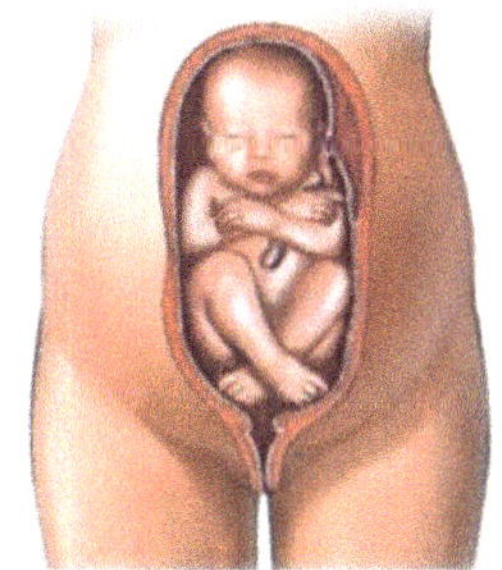
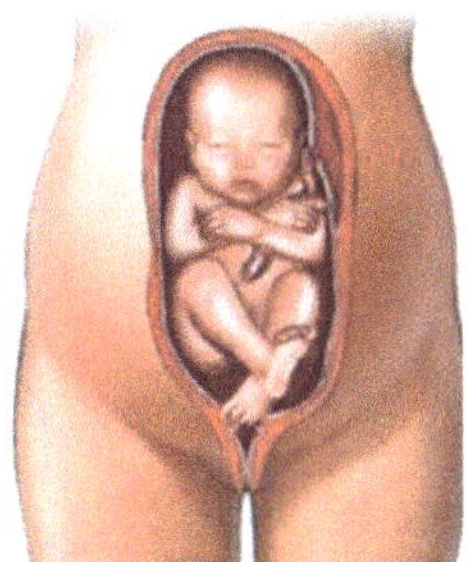

Your baby will have reached such a large size by the time you conclude your pregnancy that it will be unable to move around very much inside your womb. At this point, the majority of infants have assumed a stance in which they sit with their heads bowed. In the process of childbirth, they enter the birth canal with their heads first. When a baby is born breech, their head is protruding and they are born bottom and feet first. The birth of a baby that is breech is connected with several additional hazards and requires particular attention.

What is a Breech Baby?

As they prepare to leave your womb, the majority of newborns are in a head-down position. This particular approach, which is referred to as the vertex presentation, is the most typical. On top of that, it is the safest method for vaginal birth.

The buttocks and perhaps the feet are displayed by a newborn who is breech. A condition known as the after-coming head occurs when the bottom of the body is born first, then the body, and finally the head comes into existence last of all. An obstetrician will have a difficult time delivering a baby that is breech, and both you and your child will be at a greater risk.

Breech newborns enjoy a relatively uncomplicated neonatal phase, provided that they are delivered without incident. It does not have any impact on their growth, development, or health throughout their entire lives because they are born feet first.

Infants can also lay horizontally, in addition to lying in the vertex and breech positions. In most cases, a cesarean section is necessary to deliver a baby in this position, which is known as transverse lying.

Types of Breech Positions (Frank, Complete, Footling)

When a fetus is positioned in the uterus with its bottom or feet facing down towards the delivery canal, this is referred to as a breech baby. This is in contrast to the more frequent posture of the fetus being in the head-down (vertex) position. This location is concerned largely because it has the potential to make the delivery procedure more difficult.

There is a wide variety of breech positions, each of which has its own set of ramifications for the delivery process:

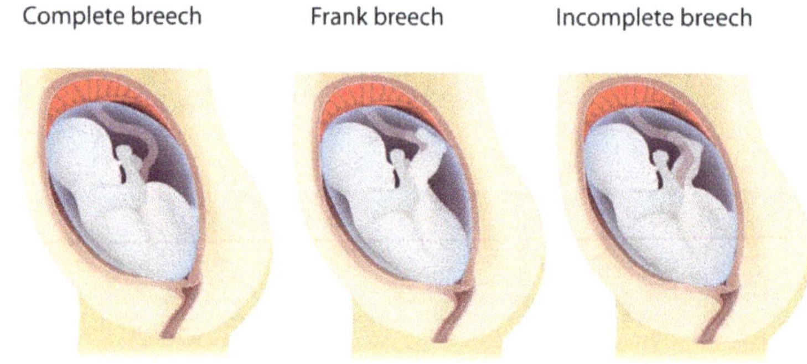

1. **Frank Breech:** The baby's buttocks are positioned to leave the body first, with the legs standing straight out in front of the body and the feet being close to the infant's head. This is the initial position of the newborn.

2. **Complete Breech**: The baby is positioned in a position known as complete breech, in which they are seated with their legs crossed, their knees and hips bowed, and their feet tucked in near to their front legs.

3. **Footling Breech:** This condition occurs when either one or both of the baby's feet are positioned to emerge first.

It is necessary to take a specialized approach to the management of the delivery process since every type of breech position has its own set of difficulties and dangers during labor and delivery.

Causes of Breech Presentation

There are a variety of factors that might cause a baby to be born in a breech position, and sometimes these factors are not completely understood.

There are, however, several elements that might contribute to this circumstance:

1. **Prematurity**: Breech presentations are more likely in preterm kids because they have not had as much time to transition into the head-down position. This is because premature babies have not yet reached full term.

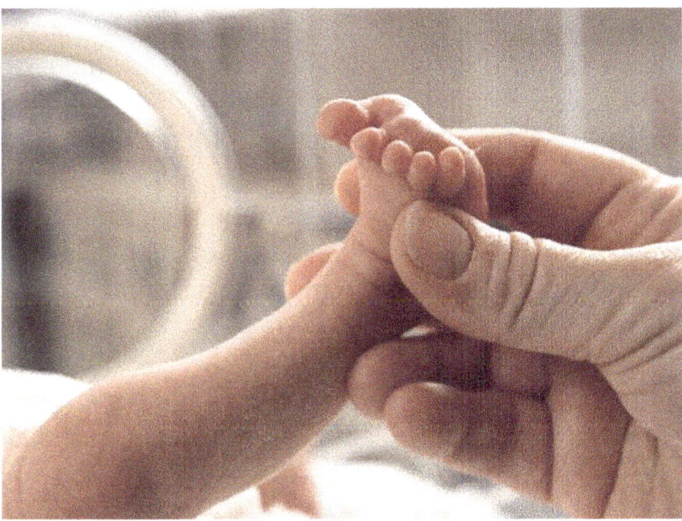

2. **Uterine Abnormalities**: Structural abnormalities in the uterus, such as fibroids or a bicornuate uterus, might hinder the baby's mobility and prevent it from going head-down. This can be a problem for the mother.

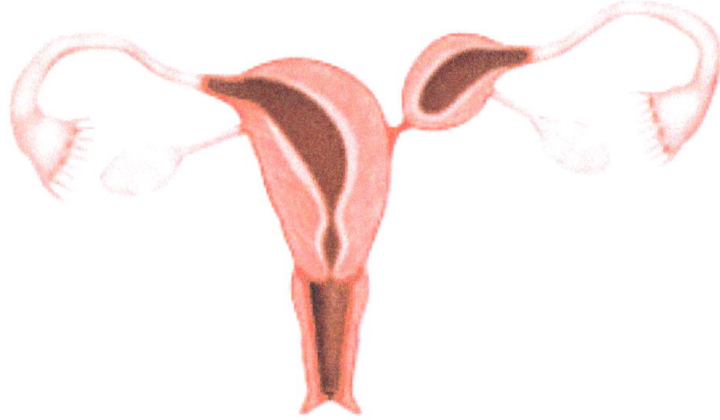

3. **Placenta Previa:** The third condition is called placenta previa, and it occurs when the placenta is situated low in the uterus. This condition might prevent the baby from shifting into the head-down position.

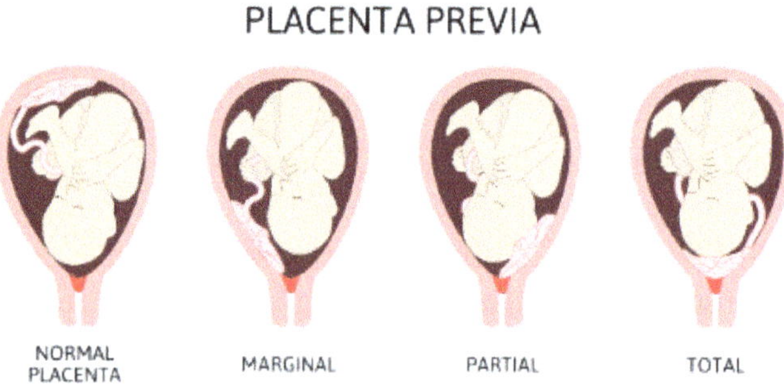

4. **Multiple Pregnancies:** In situations of twins or higher-order multiples, the room in the uterus may be restricted, which makes it more difficult for all kids to acquire a head-down position. This is specifically the case in cases where there are multiple pregnancies.

5. **Too Much or Too Little Amniotic Fluid**: An Excessive Amount of Amniotic Fluid or an Insufficient Amount of Amniotic Fluid Abnormal amounts of amniotic fluid can either provide the baby with an excessive amount of room to move or restrain their capacity to shift into the appropriate position.

It is possible for pregnant parents and their healthcare professionals to adopt a more educated and planned approach to managing breech presentation if they have a better understanding of these characteristics.

When a baby is born head-first, the hazards associated with vaginal delivery of a breech baby are less severe than those associated with head-first births. Among these dangers are the following:

1. **Prolapse of the Umbilical Cord:** This condition occurs when the umbilical cord slides into the birth canal before the baby is born. This can result in the infant being compressed and a potentially life-threatening decrease in the baby's oxygen supply.

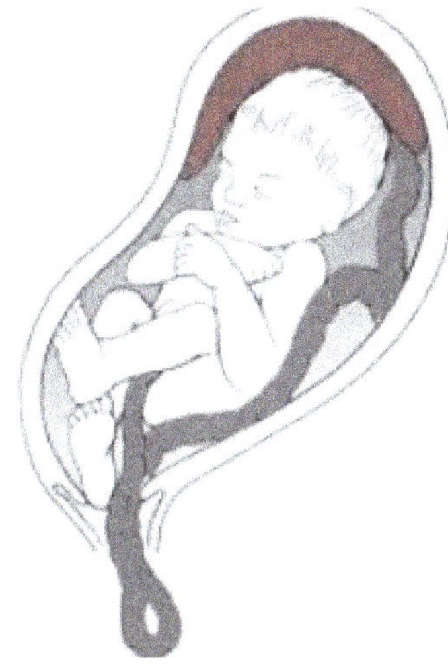

2. **Head Entrapment**: During a vaginal breech birth, the baby's body may be born before the head is, which may result in the head becoming caught. This is referred to as head entrapment.

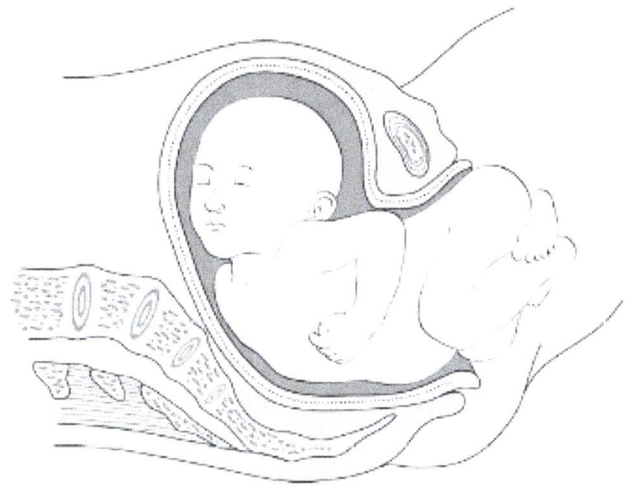

3. **Trauma and Injury:** Babies that are born breech are at a greater risk of experiencing physical injuries during birth. These injuries can include fractures, dislocations, and damage to the soft tissues.

In light of these dangers, many medical professionals advise that breech births be performed via cesarean section to provide the highest possible level of safety for both the mother and the infant. By taking the necessary precautions and making the necessary preparations, it is possible to successfully handle vaginal breech deliveries in some circumstances.

Monitoring the Position of the Fetus

During the pregnancy, it is particularly important to do regular prenatal checkups and ultrasounds to monitor the position of the fetus. In the third trimester, which occurs between 32 and 36 weeks of pregnancy, fetal position is often evaluated in great detail. If it is discovered that a newborn is lying in a breech posture, It is possible that during these evaluations, medical professionals would suggest a variety of methods and actions that will assist in turning the infant about.

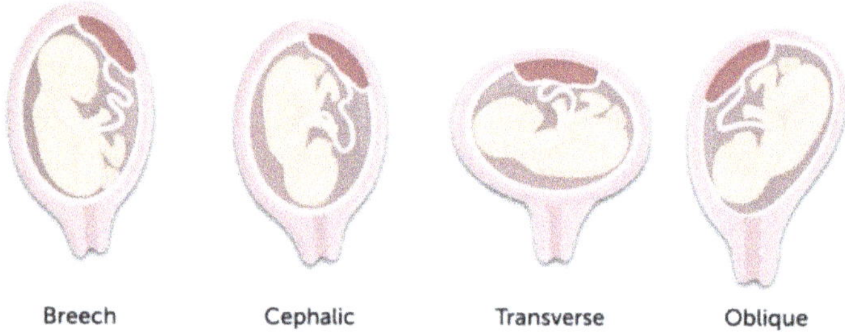

The Importance of Being Aware and Taking Action Without Delay

It is essential for pregnant parents to be aware of the breech presentation and to take action as soon as possible. Parents can take preventative measures to urge their baby to flip head-down when they have gained an awareness of the variables that lead to breech placement and the possible therapies that are available. The purpose of this book is to equip parents with the knowledge and self-assurance they need to successfully navigate this area of pregnancy.

Healthcare Providers and Their Role

Breech presentations are managed by a variety of healthcare professionals, including obstetricians, midwives, chiropractors, and other experts. These professionals play an important part in the process. In addition to providing support and assistance during the procedure, they also carry out any required medical interventions with the patient. To provide a complete and individualized strategy for turning a breech baby, parents and healthcare practitioners need to communicate well with one another.

When it comes to turning a breech baby, there are a few different methods that parents may attempt at home that do not include medical intervention. To encourage the baby to go into the head-down position, these approaches contain particular activities and positions that can be accomplished. Physical activities such as swimming, forward-leaning inversion, and pelvic tilt exercises are among the most often used approaches.

- **Exercises for the Pelvic Tilt**

The mother participates in pelvic tilt exercises by lying on her back with her hips lifted above her head.

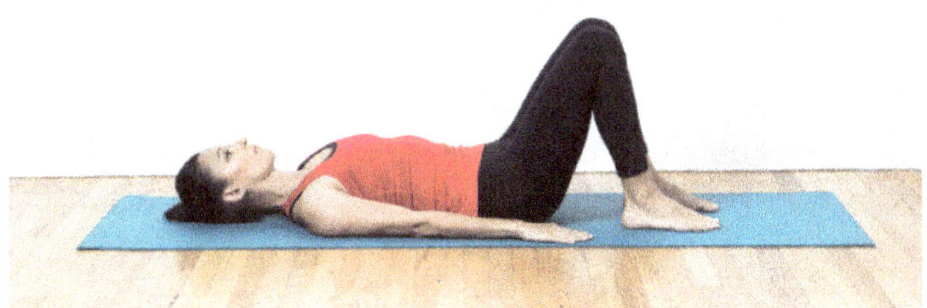

Typically, cushions are used to support her hips during these activities. The baby is encouraged to migrate out of the pelvis and maybe flip head-down when the uterus is in this position because it helps to generate more room in the bottom region of the uterus.

- **Forward-Leaning Inversion**

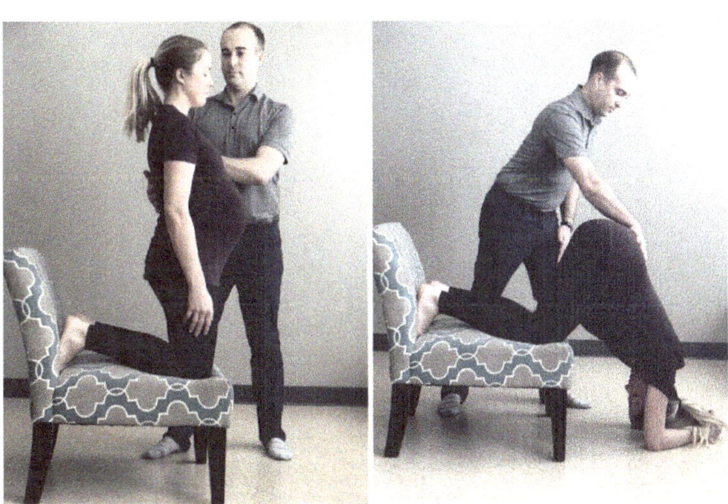

When doing the forward-leaning inversion, the mother begins by kneeling on a sofa or bed and then lowers her forearms to the floor, which results in the mother being in an inverted posture. A temporary change in the baby's position and encouragement to turn can be achieved via the use of this method.

- **Swimming**

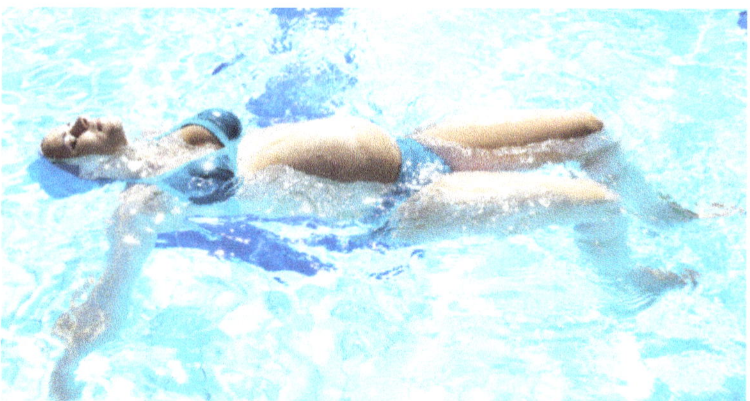

When it comes to turning a breech baby, you may find that swimming and other water workouts are effective. The buoyancy of water may assist the baby to turn in a natural manner since it will aid in alleviating the pressure that is being applied to the infant and will make movement easier.

Medical Interventions for Turning Breech Babies

Healthcare experts can prescribe medical procedures such as the External Cephalic Version (ECV), chiropractic techniques such as the Webster technique, or alternative therapies such as acupuncture and moxibustion in situations when non-medical techniques do not prove to be helpful.

- **"External Cephalic Version" (ECV)**

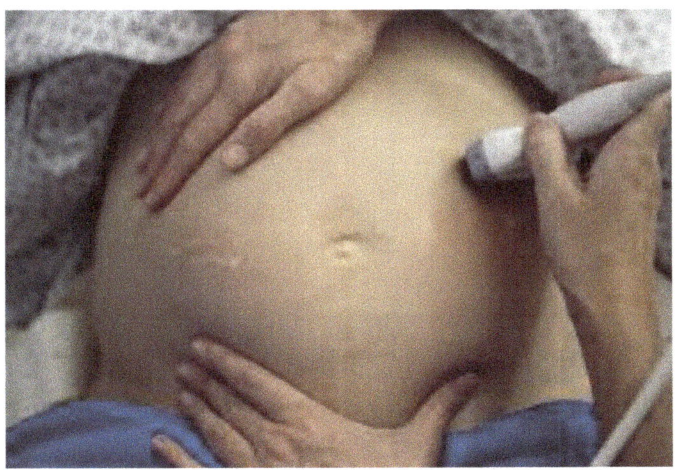

During the 36th to 37th week of pregnancy, an obstetrician would often conduct an ECV operation in a hospital environment. This surgery is performed by an obstetrician. The physician will apply pressure to the mother's belly to attempt to flip the baby from the outside while the surgery is being performed. Although ECV has the potential to be helpful, it is not appropriate for all pregnancies and comes with many dangers.

- **Chiropractic Techniques (Webster Technique)**

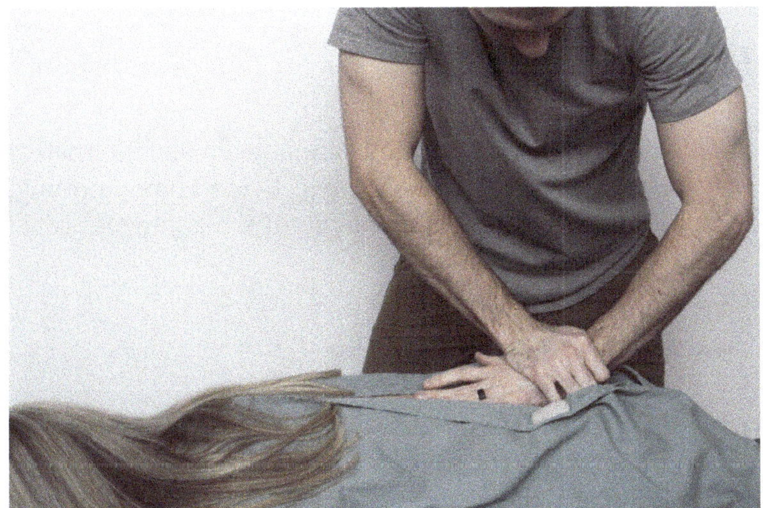

The Webster technique is a chiropractic approach that was developed to relieve tension in the uterus and bring the pelvis into proper alignment. By utilizing this method, additional room may be created for the infant to roam about and possibly turn their head down. During pregnancy, it is essential to choose a chiropractor who has prior experience working with women who are pregnant.

- **Acupuncture and Moxibustion**

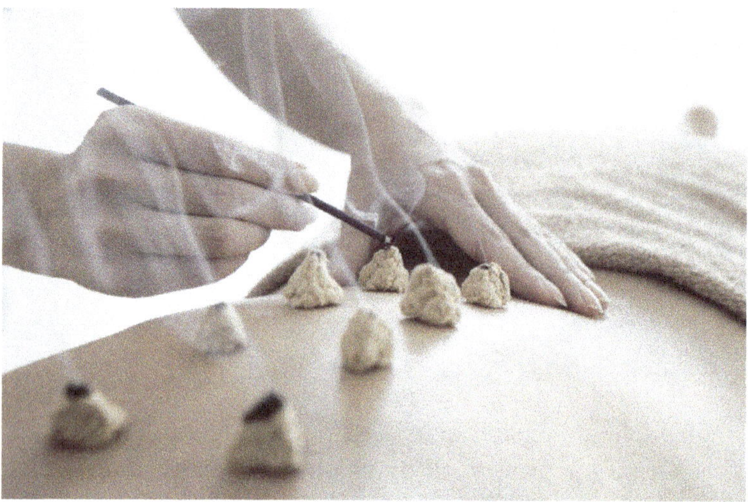

Acupuncture and moxibustion are two of the various methods that are available in traditional Chinese medicine for turning breech newborns. Moxibustion is a technique that includes burning a herb near certain locations on the body to induce movement, whereas acupuncture involves placing small needles into specific sites on the physical body. Both of these methods are helpful in clinical research, and their primary objective is to urge the baby to turn over.

Alternative and Holistic Methods

In addition to the approaches described above, several other methods are holistic and alternative that parents may investigate to assist their breech baby in turning over. Hypnobirthing, visualization, talking to the baby, and the use of heat and cold are some of the approaches that fall under this category.

- **Birthing with Hypnosis and Visualization**

Hypnobirthing is a method of giving birth that incorporates the use of relaxation and visualization methods to generate a peaceful and optimistic state of mind, which can affect the position of the baby. Visualization is a technique that includes mentally imagining the baby laying over with its head down. This technique can be used with deep relaxation techniques.

- **Talking to the Baby**

It has been shown that chatting to one's infant and gently coaxing them to roll over might be beneficial for certain households. When music is played toward the bottom area of the belly, it may also encourage the baby to move closer to the sound rather than away from it.

- **Applying both heat and cold**

By applying heat to the lower belly and cold to the upper abdomen, it is possible to occasionally urge the baby to migrate toward the warmth and away from the cold. It is essential to make use of methods that are both safe and delicate while administering heat and cold to prevent any discomfort or injury from occurring.

Problem-Solving and Troubleshooting

Not every breech baby will flip over to face down, despite the greatest efforts of the parents. It is essential for parents to realize that they have exercised their best efforts and to investigate alternate birth plans if they are required to do so. It is also essential to learn how to manage anxiety and stress, since having a calm and optimistic mentality may have an effect on the birthing experience as a whole.

When Methods Do Not Produce the Desired Results

Parents need to explore alternate birth plans with their healthcare practitioner if non-medical approaches and medical treatments do not prove to be beneficial. An example of this would be making arrangements for a cesarean section or getting ready for a vaginal breech delivery, if the latter is considered to be safe.

Methods for Handling Stress and Anxiety

Both pregnancy and labor may be emotional and stressful experiences, particularly when difficulties such as breech presentation occur. When it comes to managing anxiety and stress, parents need to discover ways to cope with these emotions. Included in this category are the utilization of relaxation methods and mindfulness practices, as well as the solicitation of support from partners, family members, and friends.

Acquiring Knowledge of Medical Advice

To comprehend medical advice and make well-informed decisions, maintaining consistent communication with healthcare experts is crucial. Any concerns that parents may have regarding breech presentation and delivery choices should be addressed in a manner that allows them to feel at ease asking questions and seeking clarity.

Exceptional Circumstances and Important Ideas

Some circumstances call for additional considerations and measures, such as having many pregnancies, having multiple breech deliveries in the past, and having a high-risk pregnancy. Parents who find themselves in these circumstances should make it a priority to collaborate closely with their healthcare professionals to devise a bespoke strategy for the management of breech presentation.

Having more than one child

When there are multiples of a higher order or twins, the space in the uterus may be restricted, which makes it more challenging for all of the kids to be in a position where they are with their heads down. The management of breech presentation in multiple pregnancies may necessitate the use of certain procedures and medical measures.

Earlier births that were breech

There is a possibility that parents who have already had a breech delivery would have distinct worries and requirements. The management of breech presentation in successive pregnancies can be achieved by the application of approaches that are tailored to the individual's personal history and the learning from previous experiences.

High-Risk Pregnancies

When a woman is carrying a high-risk pregnancy, she must take additional care and make modifications to ensure that both she and her unborn child remain safe. In situations like these, conducting close collaboration with healthcare practitioners and specialists is necessary to devise a method that is both safe and successful for treating breech presentation.

Post-Turn Care and Follow-Up

It is essential to keep a close eye on the position of a breech baby once they have successfully turned their head down. This will allow you to be ready for labor and delivery. To guarantee that the baby continues to be in the head-down position, it is important to have routine checkups and ultrasounds.

Monitoring Following a Turn That Was Successful

Following a successful turnaround, medical professionals will continue to keep a close eye on the baby's position to make sure it continues to be in the head-down position. This may include routine checkups and ultrasounds.

Preparing for the Birthing Process and Labor

As part of the last preparations for labor and delivery, you will need to pack your belongings for the hospital or birth center and collaborate with your healthcare specialists to negotiate the birth plan. It is essential to have a flexible approach to the birthing process and to be ready for a variety of different circumstances.

When a baby is born breech, the process of flipping them over might be difficult, but it also presents a chance for personal development and education. Sharing the tale with others and reflecting on the experience can give significant insights and support for other expectant parents who are going through issues that are similar to those that you have been through.

CHAPTER ONE

Basics of Breech Presentation

Anatomy of Pregnancy

To know the reasons and mechanisms behind breech presentations, it is essential to have a fundamental understanding of the anatomy of pregnancy. During pregnancy, the uterus, which is shaped like a pear and is located in the pelvis, is the organ that contributes to the growth of the baby. Three primary components make up the uterus: the fundus, which is located at the top, the body, which is located in the center, and the cervix, which is located at the bottom and opens into the vagina.

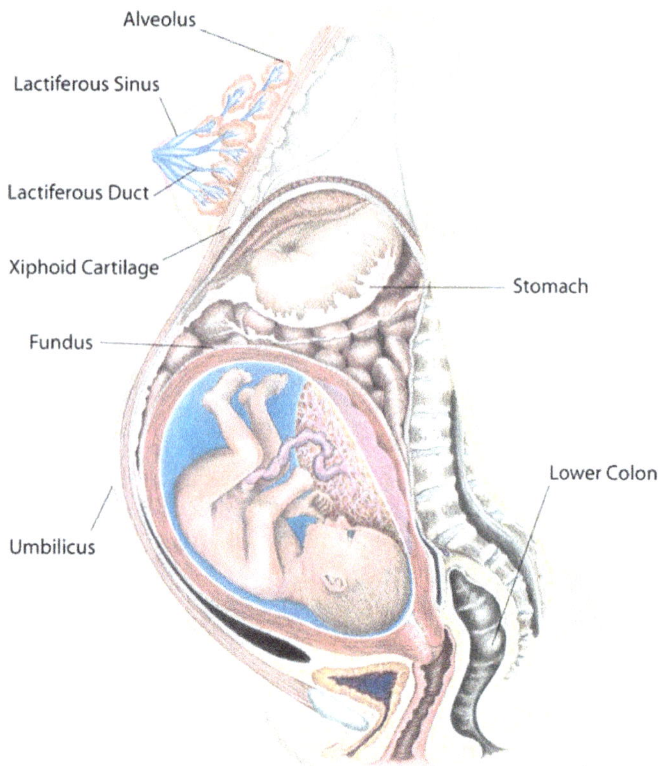

Throughout pregnancy, the position of the baby within the uterus might become dramatically different. During the early stages of pregnancy, the baby has plenty of room to move around and can regularly switch positions. However, during the third trimester, the baby has grown greatly, and the room has become restricted, which results in the baby being positioned more stably.

Around the 32nd to 36th week of pregnancy, a typical full-term fetus should have reached the optimal posture of settling into a head-down position, also known as the vertex position. The head, which is the biggest component of the infant, can go through the birth canal first when the baby is in this position. This is the safest and most effective approach to deliver a baby through the vaginal route. On the other hand, the baby stays in a breech position in around three to four percent of pregnancies. An in-depth investigation of the elements that influence fetal placement is required to have an understanding of why this occurs.

How Babies Turn in the Womb

During pregnancy, particularly during the third trimester, it is common for expecting mothers to arrange their newborns in a head-down position in preparation for delivery. During this part of the pregnancy, which is referred to as "**engagement**," the head of the baby moves down into the pelvis. This typically occurs between the 34th and 36th week of pregnancy. Several elements contribute to the natural turning process, including the following:

- **Amniotic Fluid**: The amount of amniotic fluid in the uterus affects the degree to which the baby can move about. The ability of the baby to turn can be hindered by either an inadequate amount of fluid (oligohydramnios) or an excessive amount of fluid (polyhydramnios). Adequate fluid allows for easier mobility.

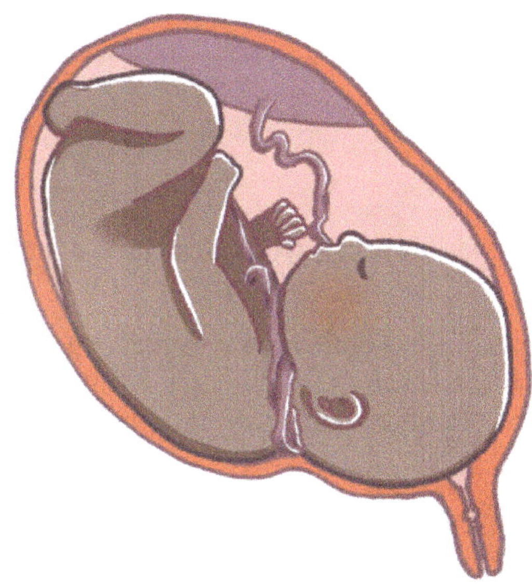

- **Uterine Shape:** The size and shape of the uterus, which can be affected by variables such as uterine abnormalities (for example, a bicornuate uterus) or the presence of fibroids, can affect the movement and placement of the fetus.

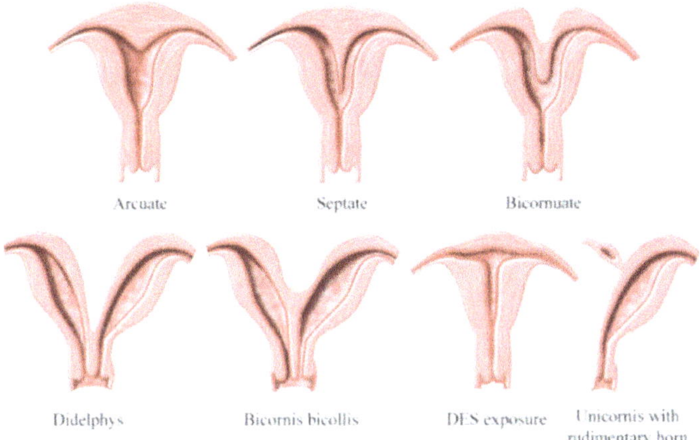

- **Fetal Activity:** Babies are naturally active while they are still within the mother's womb, and the fetal movement plays a key influence in deciding where they are located. As they develop, they investigate the space that is accessible to them, which ultimately determines where they will be when they are born.

- **Changing postures and Activities of the Mother:** The movements, postures, and activities of the mother can also have an effect on the position of the baby after birth. Two factors might either promote or prevent the baby from going into a head-down position: gravity and the posture of the mother.

When and How Breech Positions are Diagnosed

The identification of breech situations often takes place during normal prenatal appointments, particularly during the third trimester of pregnancy.

A breech presentation can be diagnosed using a variety of approaches, including the following:

- **Palpation**: When performing a physical examination, medical professionals are frequently able to establish the position of the baby by feeling the position of the mother's belly. The head, buttocks, and limbs of the infant each have their unique sensations that may be differentiated by expert hands.

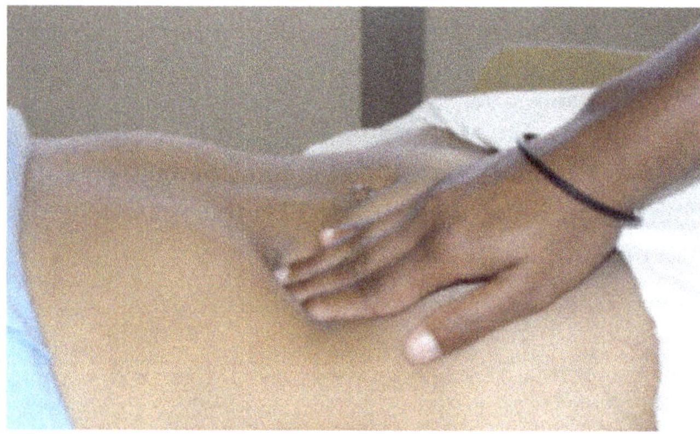

- **Ultrasound**: Breech presentation can be diagnosed with more accuracy using ultrasound imaging, which is a more advanced technique. It enables medical professionals to visually confirm the location of the baby and check for any potential issues that may require attention.

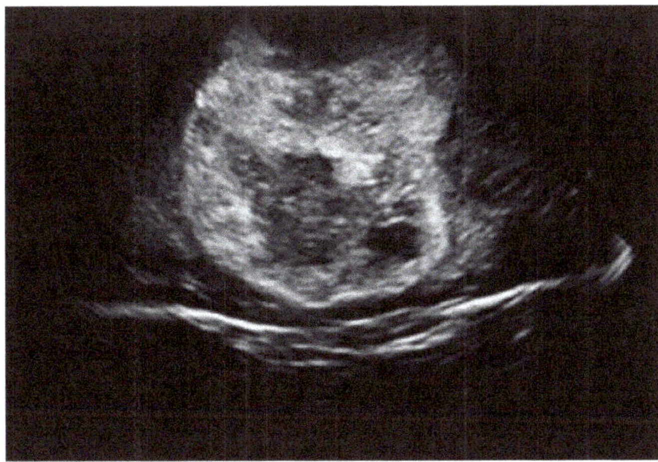

- **Leopold Maneuvers:** This particular sequence of four procedures entails palpating the belly of the mother to ascertain the position, presentation, and engagement of the baby in the pelvis.

- **Fetal Heart Tones:** The direction in which the strongest fetal heart tones are heard might offer information regarding the position of the baby. While heart tones are often heard below the umbilicus of the mother when the baby is in the vertex position, they are typically heard above the umbilicus when the baby is in the breech position.

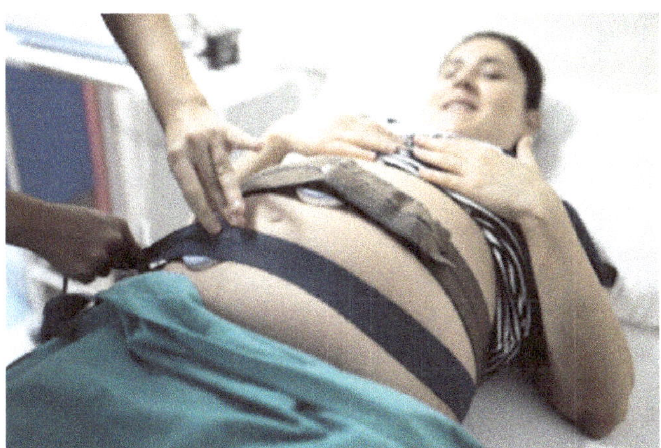

Typically, the diagnosis takes place around the 36th week of pregnancy, which is also the time when the position of the baby becomes increasingly important for determining the manner of infant birth. It is frequently important to conduct additional monitoring and evaluation if a breach location is identified.

Monitoring the Position of the Fetus

After a diagnosis of breech presentation has been made, it is necessary to do continuous monitoring to keep track of the baby's position and to make educated decisions regarding delivery.

As part of this monitoring, we will:

- **Follow-Up Ultrasounds**: It is possible to arrange regular ultrasounds to determine whether or not the baby has turned over, as well as to assess the amounts of amniotic fluid and the location of the placenta.

- **Non-Stress tests (NSTs):** The purpose of non-stress tests, also known as NSTs, is to ensure that the baby is healthy and not under any kind of stress by monitoring the baby's heart rate and movements.

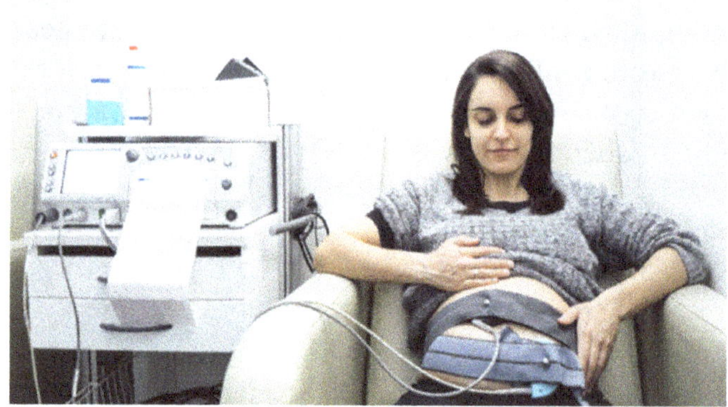

- **Biophysical Profile (BPP):** The Biophysical Profile (BPP) is a thorough examination that combines an ultrasound and a non-stress test (NST) to measure the level of amniotic fluid, the movements of the baby, the tone of the baby's muscles, and the baby's breathing motions.

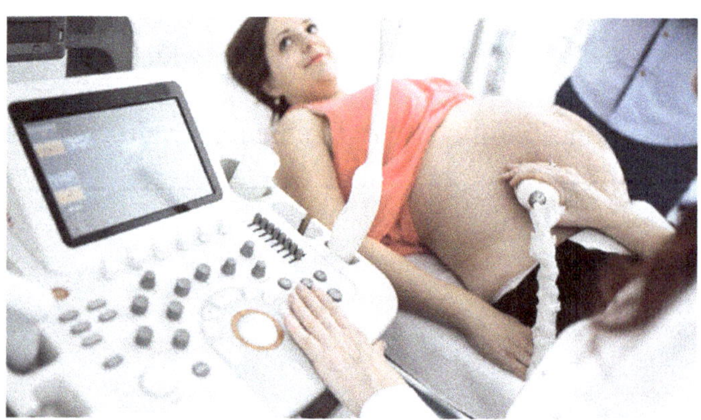

- **Pelvic Examinations**: In the later stages of pregnancy, pelvic examinations can help determine the position of the baby and the degree to which the baby is engaged in the pelvis.

Close monitoring enables medical professionals to determine the chance of a spontaneous turn occurring and to make preparations for either an attempt to turn the baby or for a safe delivery strategy, which may include a cesarean section or a vaginal birth.

CHAPTER TWO

Understanding Your Options

Handling a breech baby during pregnancy can be difficult and stressful. It is essential to know your alternatives to make well-informed selections that best fit your unique situation and medical requirements. This chapter explores the many options available to you, their benefits and drawbacks, how to communicate effectively with your healthcare professional, and how to get ready both physically and psychologically for the results.

Vaginal Breech Birth vs. Cesarean Section

The two main methods for delivering a breech baby are cesarean surgery (C-section) and vaginal breech delivery. Every technique has advantages and disadvantages of its own, and the choice is frequently influenced by many variables like the mother's health, the baby's size, the kind of breech presentation, and the healthcare provider's expertise.

Vaginal Breech Birth

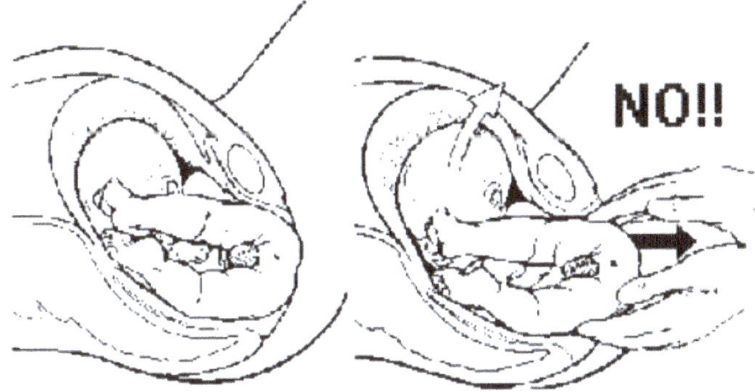

Vaginal breech births were more prevalent in the past, but as medical research has advanced and worries about the hazards of breech deliveries have grown, many healthcare practitioners now prefer cesarean sections. On the other hand, a vaginal breech delivery might be a safe alternative under specific situations.

Benefits:

- **Shorter Recovery Time:** Compared to C-sections, vaginal deliveries typically result in shorter hospital stays and speedier recoveries.

- **Lower Risk of Surgical Complications**: Refusing major surgery lowers the chance of developing blood clots, infections, and anesthesia-related side effects.

- **Instant Bonding and nursing**: When a baby is delivered vaginally, it's common to lay them right on the mother's chest, which encourages instant bonding and nursing.

Cons:

- **Greater Risk of Trauma**: Breech newborns are more likely to sustain physical trauma during vaginal birth, including soft tissue damage, fractures, and dislocations.

- **Umbilical cord Prolapse**: In this situation, the umbilical cord may prolapse into the delivery canal before the infant, perhaps severing their oxygen supply.

- **Head Entrapment:** The baby's body can be delivered before the head, which might cause entrapment and make delivery challenging.

C-section, or cesarean section

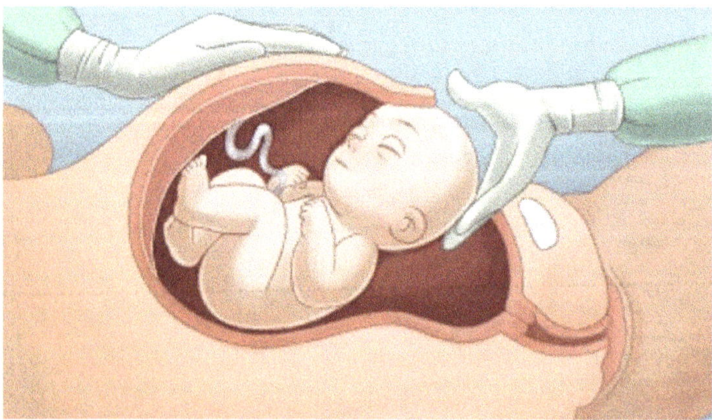

A C-section is a surgical operation in which the mother's abdomen and uterus are cut open to deliver the baby. For breech deliveries, this technique is frequently advised to reduce the dangers involved with vaginal delivery.

Advantages:

- **Controlled Environment:** Since a C-section is a scheduled, regulated operation, the likelihood of a breech vaginal delivery is decreased.

- **Lower Risk of Birth Trauma**: Compared to vaginal breech births, there is a far smaller chance that the infant may sustain physical damage during birth.

- **Lower Risk of Head Entrapment and Umbilical Cord Prolapse**: A C-section almost eliminates these problems.

Cons:

- **Lengthier healing Period:** Compared to vaginal births, healing following a C-section is more complicated and requires longer hospital stays and recovery times.

- **Enhanced Risk of Surgical problems**: C-sections are more likely to result in infections, blood clots, and anesthesia-related problems than other major surgeries.

- **Effect on Subsequent Pregnancies:** Placenta previa and uterine rupture are two issues that may arise from a C-section.

Added Pros and Cons of Different Birth Plans

Weighing the benefits and drawbacks of a vaginal delivery against a cesarean section is necessary to choose the optimal birth plan for a breech baby. Here's a closer look at the factors to think about with each choice:

Vaginal Breech Birth

Advantages:

- **Natural delivery Experience**: The instant bonding that results from a natural delivery is something that many moms find appealing.

- **Lower Healthcare Costs**: Medical costs associated with vaginal deliveries are often lower than those associated with surgical births.

- **Faster Postpartum Recovery**: Following vaginal deliveries, women frequently recover more rapidly, enduring less pain and fewer difficulties during the postpartum phase.

Cons:

- **Experienced practitioner Needed**: Not all hospitals may have a professional and experienced healthcare practitioner on staff, which is necessary for a successful vaginal breech delivery.

- **Greater Risk of Emergency C-Section**: An emergency C-section, which can be more stressful and dangerous than a scheduled C-section, may be required if difficulties occur during a vaginal breech birth.

Cesarean Section

Pros:

- **Predictability and Planning:** By allowing parents to make plans for the delivery, a planned C-section lowers anxiety and uncertainty.

- **Controlled Environment**: Managing breech deliveries can benefit greatly from the controlled environment that the surgical setting offers.

Cons:

- **Extended Hospital Stay**: Postoperative treatment following a C-section usually involves a lengthier hospital stay.

- **Physical and Emotional Impact**: If a woman had hoped for a vaginal delivery, she may feel let down by the longer and more painful physical recovery following a C-section.

Selecting the optimal method for delivering a breech baby requires effective communication between you and your healthcare professional. The following tactics can help to guarantee fruitful conversations:

Preparing for the Conversation

- **Conduct Research**: Recognize the fundamentals of breech presentation and the available delivery options. This will enable you to comprehend the information your healthcare practitioner is providing and to ask thoughtful questions.

- **Create a list of inquiries**: Make a note of the queries and worries you want to address with your healthcare professional. This might involve inquiring about the advantages and disadvantages of every delivery technique, their expertise with breech deliveries, and the facilities and policies of the hospital.

Important Questions to Ask

- **Training and Experience**: "What is your level of experience with handling breech births? What kind of training have you had for vaginal breech births?"

- **Dangers and Success Rates:** "What are the success rates and risks associated with vaginal breech birth and C-section in your practice?"

- **Hospital Policies**: "What are the policies regarding breech births at the hospital? Do any particular guidelines or restrictions exist?"

- **Emergency Procedures**: "What would happen if a vaginal breech delivery encounters difficulties? How soon can a C-section be performed in an emergency?

Understanding the Answers

- **Clarify Medical Jargon**: Never be afraid to seek clarification on any medical jargon or procedures you are unsure about. You must have complete knowledge of your available alternatives.

- **Get Second Opinions**: You should think about getting a second opinion from a different medical professional or expert if you have doubts about the guidance you've been given.

Preparing Mentally and Physically for Different Scenarios

Managing the uncertainty and worry that might accompany a breech pregnancy requires preparation.

The following techniques can be used to emotionally and physically get ready for both a cesarean surgery and a vaginal breech birth:

Mental Readiness

- **Become Informed:** Acquiring knowledge gives one strength. Learn more about breech births and your alternatives for delivery by reading books, going to workshops, and joining support groups.

- **Show Off Your Success**: Using visualization methods might assist you in psychologically preparing for a successful delivery. Imagine that you have delivered your kid safely and are holding them for the first time.

- **Mindfulness and Relaxation**: To reduce stress and keep a good outlook, engage in mindfulness, meditation, and relaxation techniques. Particularly helpful methods include gradual muscle relaxation, deep breathing, and prenatal yoga.

Physical Preparation

- **Remain Active**: You may enhance your strength, flexibility, and general wellbeing by engaging in regular exercise throughout pregnancy. Prenatal yoga, swimming, and walking are all excellent choices.

- **Exercises for the Pelvic Floor:** These, along with other positioning methods, can help your body become ready for birth. For advice on the appropriate workouts for your circumstances, speak with a physical therapist or your healthcare practitioner.

- **Nutrition and Hydration**: Eat a balanced diet and drink plenty of water. Eating a healthy diet helps your body meet the demands of becoming pregnant and giving birth.

- **Get Ready for Postpartum Recovery**: Be ready for the postpartum phase whether you're having a C-section or a vaginal birth. Stock up on vital supplies, organize for help with domestic responsibilities, and prepare for relaxation and recuperation.

Creating a Birth Plan

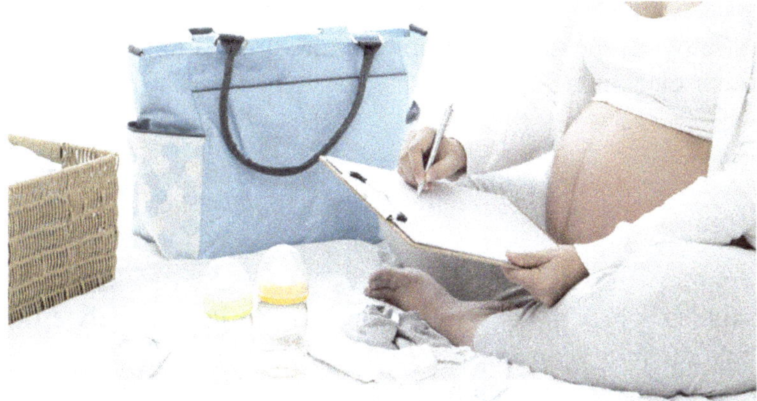

Making a birth plan can give you a sense of control and readiness for a variety of situations. Your choices for pain management, support systems, and any other unique demands you may have for the birthing process are all outlined in your birth plan.

What to include is as follows:

- **Personal Details**: Contact details, name, and deadline.

- **Labor Preferences:** Preferences regarding pain management, mobility, and labor jobs.

- **Delivery Preferences**: Choices about episiotomy, forceps or vacuum delivery, and vaginal or C-section birth.

- **Post-Delivery Care**: Arrangements for nursing, newborn care, and instant skin-to-skin contact.

- **Contingency Plans:** What to do if unanticipated difficulties arise or the birth plan is altered.

CHAPTER THREE

Non-Medical Techniques for Turning Breech Babies (Beginner Level)

Finding out that your baby is breech might be one of the many twists and shocks that come with being pregnant. The methods covered in this chapter are non-medical and can be used at home by pregnant parents to assist their breech baby in turning to the head-down position, which is optimal for a vaginal birth. There's no need for medical involvement to try these approaches; they are typically safe.

This chapter covers several important strategies, including swimming, forward-leaning inversion, pelvic tilt exercises, and advice for mother placement.

Pelvic Tilt Exercises

Simple yet effective techniques for assisting a breech baby to flip head-down include pelvic tilt exercises. With these activities, you may encourage the baby to turn from the breech position by arranging your body to create more room in the bottom region of the uterus.

The process:

Preparation

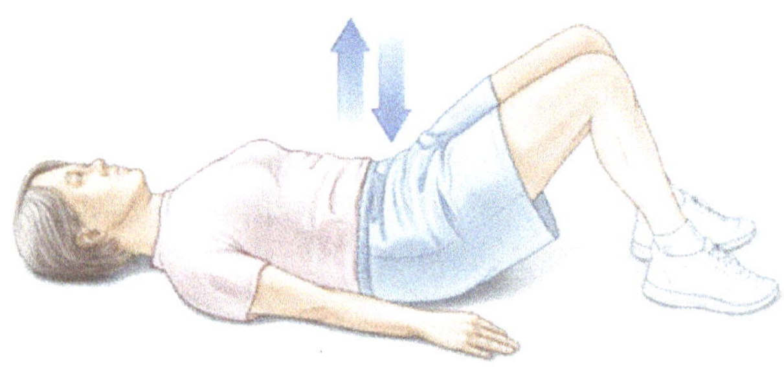

- Look for a peaceful, comfortable area where you may do the activity without being disturbed. For extra comfort, you might require a yoga mat or a carpeted space.

- Make sure you have cushions or pillows handy to support your hips and back.

Positioning

- Rest on your back, legs bent, and feet flat on the ground.

- To raise your pelvis, place one or two cushions beneath your hips. There should be an inclination where your hips and shoulders meet.

Execution

- Breathe slowly and deeply while reclining your arms by your sides.

- Hold this posture for ten to fifteen minutes, letting the baby's natural movement out of the pelvis and maybe head-down be encouraged by gravity.

Frequency

- For optimal effects, perform this exercise two to three times each day. Being consistent is essential for promoting mobility.

Benefits and Precautions

Benefits:

- You can practice this workout at home and it's quite easy.

- It encourages relaxation and gives expecting moms a chance to connect with their bodies and babies.

- It helps generate more room in the lower uterus, which can encourage the baby to shift into the head-down position.

Precautions:

- Do not perform this exercise if you are in pain, uncomfortable, or lightheaded.

- Before beginning this activity, especially if you have any problems or health issues, speak with your healthcare professional.

- Use cushions to offer sufficient support and avoid straining your neck and back.

Forward-Leaning Inversion

Another useful method for aiding a breech infant in turning is the forward-leaning inversion. By inverting the body during this exercise, you can momentarily change the baby's posture and urge it to turn head-down.

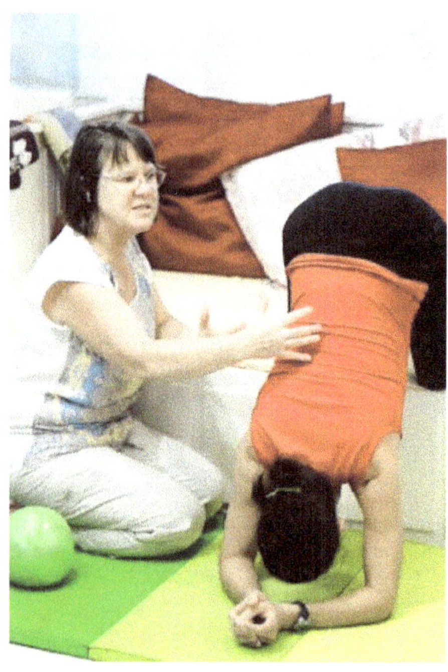

How to Work Safely

Preparation

- Select a safe place to kneel, such as a couch or bed, that is firm and secure.

- Make sure there are no obstructions in the way to avoid accidents or falls.

Positioning

- Place your knees hip-width apart on the edge of the bed or sofa.

- Lower your forearms gradually so that your head rests on the ground. An inverted posture is achieved when your hips are higher than your shoulders.

Execution

- Focus on taking calm, deep breaths while holding this position for 30 to 1 minute.

- Carefully stand back up straight, being careful not to move too quickly or suddenly.

Frequency

- Do this workout once or twice a day. As you get more accustomed to the posture, gradually extend the duration.

Advantages and Precautions

Advantages:

- The baby's posture is briefly altered by this activity, which facilitates head-down positioning.

- It improves attention and relaxation; it can release tension in the hips and lower back and promote flexibility.

Precautions

- To avoid falls or injuries, do this exercise only on a sturdy surface.

- If you are dizzy, have high blood pressure, or have any other medical condition that might be made worse by inversion, stay away from this activity.

- Before beginning this activity, be sure it is safe for your particular condition by speaking with your healthcare physician.

Swimming and Water Exercises

A breech infant can be gently and successfully turned by swimming. Water's buoyancy makes moving simpler for the baby and relieves pressure points, both of which might encourage rotation.

Movement Types

1. **Freestyle Swimming:**

- A baby may be encouraged to move by swimming in a front crawl or freestyle posture, which produces a little rocking motion.

- Pay attention to keeping a calm and even cadence.

2. **Backstroke:**

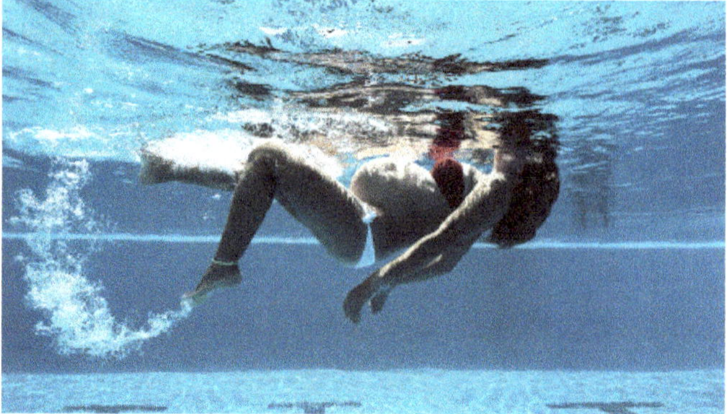

- The buoyancy of the water supports your body as you swim on your back, allowing you to unwind and take deep breaths.

- By making room in the lower uterus, this posture may encourage the baby to turn.

3. **Water Walking:**

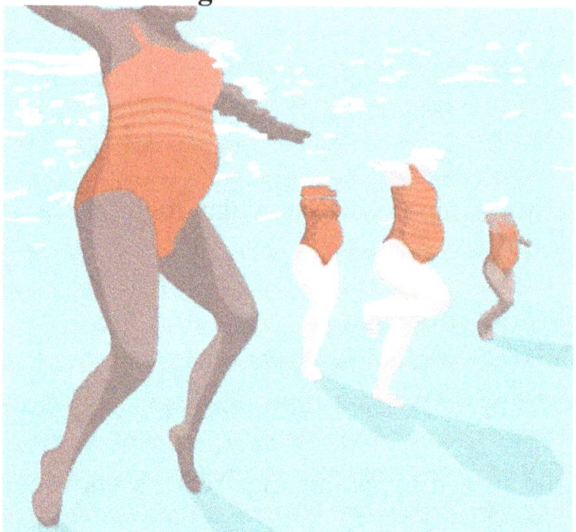

- Walking in water that is waist-deep promotes pelvic mobility and offers mild resistance.

- Pay attention to keeping your posture straight and walking at a steady, deliberate pace.

Benefits of Buoyancy

Benefits:

- The body is supported by the buoyancy of water, which lessens the stress on joints and muscles.

- Water resistance offers a mild workout, enhancing general fitness and flexibility; swimming and water workouts encourage relaxation and stress alleviation.

Precautions:

- Steer clear of swimming in water that is too hot or cold.

- To avoid getting tired, drink plenty of water and take pauses as required.

- Before beginning any water workout program, especially if you have any medical concerns or difficulties, speak with your healthcare physician.

Maternal Positioning Tips

Apart from particular activities, including certain advice for maternal posture in everyday routines might aid in encouraging a breech baby to turn. The ideal setting for the infant to transition into the head-down position is produced by these positions.

Ideal Positions to Promote Turning

1. **Pose on your hands and knees:**
- Take some time to pose with your tummy hanging down. This posture stimulates the baby to shift head-down and helps to make room in the uterus.

- For comfort, use a cushioned surface or yoga mat.

2. **Sitting on an Exercise Ball:**

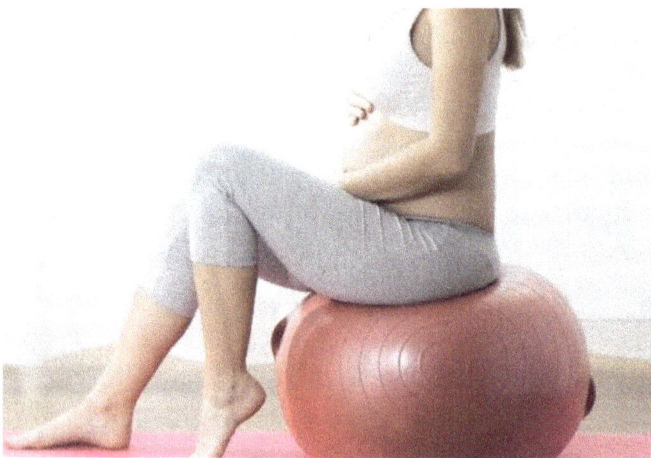

- Place your feet flat on the ground and your knees hip-width apart while sitting on an exercise ball.

- Rock your hips gently side to side and back and forth. This motion facilitates the opening of the pelvis, allowing the baby to turn comfortably.

3. **Hip Elevation:**

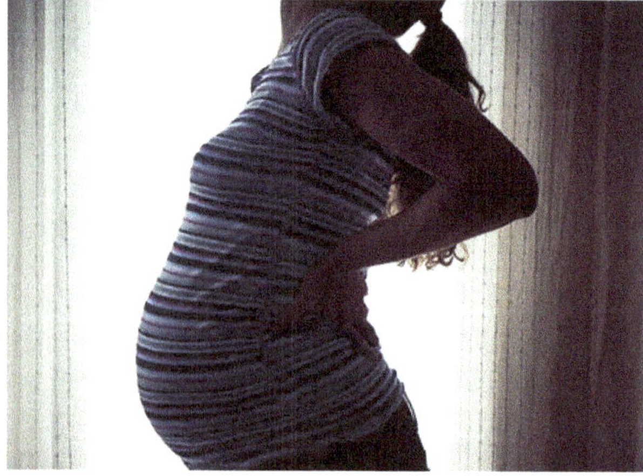

- While lying on your side, lay a cushion or pillow beneath your hips to raise them just a little.

- The baby's weight is shifted and twisting is encouraged in this position.

Daily Schedules and Habits

1. **Avoid Reclining**: Try to keep your posture upright, especially when sitting for extended periods. Rather, sit up straight with your hips slightly forward and your back straight.

2. **Remain Active**: Frequent exercise, including walking or prenatal yoga, helps support the baby's ideal posture by maintaining the pelvis' flexibility.

3. **Mindful Movement:** Throughout the day, be aware of your posture and movements. Steer clear of sitting in ways that impede pelvic mobility, such as crossing your legs.

Benefits and Precautions

Benefits:

- Keeping an active lifestyle and maintaining proper posture helps enhance overall comfort and well-being throughout pregnancy.

- These positioning guidelines are simple to implement into everyday routines and assist in creating an ideal environment for the baby to turn its head down.

Precautions:

- Steer clear of painful or uncomfortable situations.

- Pay attention to your body and take pauses as required.

- Before beginning a new fitness regimen or making major adjustments to your daily schedule, speak with your healthcare physician.

CHAPTER FOUR

Medical Interventions (Advanced Level)

When home cures and non-medical treatments are ineffective in turning a breech infant to the head-down position, medical procedures become critical. To induce a breech baby to turn, advanced medical procedures, carried out by healthcare experts, offer more regulated and supervised techniques.

This chapter explores several medical procedures, such as the External Cephalic Version (ECV), the Webster Technique in chiropractic care, and acupuncture and moxibustion as alternative remedies. Each section offers thorough explanations of various techniques, including their advantages, disadvantages, and procedural specifics.

External Cephalic Version (ECV)

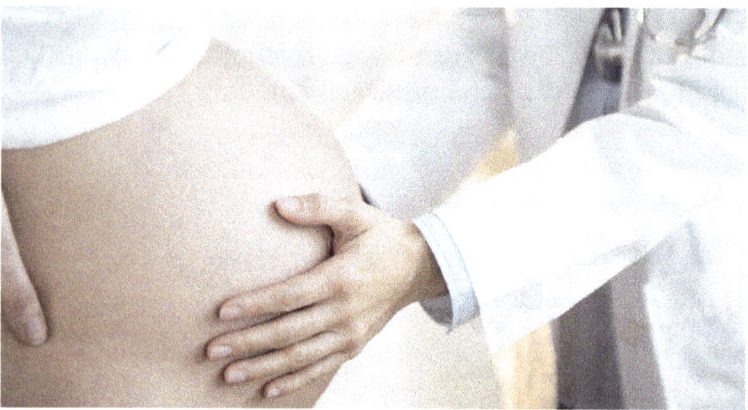

When a baby is a breech, one of the most often advised and used medical procedures is the External Cephalic Version (ECV). To promote a head-down (vertex) posture, the fetus is manually moved through the mother's abdominal wall during an ECV. Although it can be tried up to the start of labor, this treatment is usually carried out during the 36th or 37th week of pregnancy.

Detailed Description of the Process

The ECV method is often performed in a hospital setting to guarantee that emergency medical assistance is available.

This is a detailed breakdown of the steps involved in doing ECV:

1. **Preparation**

- **Assessment**: The medical professional does a comprehensive examination of the mother and child, which includes an ultrasound to verify the baby's position, the volume of amniotic fluid, and the placenta's location.

- **Informed Consent**: The mother is told about the operation, its advantages, dangers, and available options before giving her assent.

- **Fetal Monitoring:** Throughout the process, the baby's heart rate is tracked and its wellbeing is guaranteed with the use of continuous fetal monitoring.

2. **Positioning:**

- The mother is positioned such that she is comfortable; she often lies on her back with her head slightly raised. A little inclination to the left or right can help to maximize uterine position and increase comfort.

3. **Medication Administration:**

- To relax the uterus and lessen contractions, a tocolytic drug like terbutaline may be given. This will make it simpler to flip the baby.

4. **Manual Manipulation:**

- The medical professional uses both hands to gently turn the infant by applying forceful yet moderate pressure to the mother's abdomen. Usually, one hand is put on the baby's head while the other is placed on the infant's back or butt.

- The caregiver tries to turn the infant into a head-down posture by guiding it into a forward or backward somersault.

5. **Monitoring and Assessment:**

- Throughout the process, the baby's position and heart rate are continually checked. The process is stopped right away if the infant exhibits any indications of discomfort.

- A further ultrasound is carried out following the surgery to verify the baby's new location.

6. **Post-Procedure Care:**

- A brief time of observation is spent with the mother to make sure no problems, including labor or placental abruption, occur. Until the baby's well being is verified, fetal monitoring is continued.

Risks and Success Rates

Success Rates

The mother's parity (whether she has given birth previously), the baby's position, the amount of amniotic fluid, and the practitioner's expertise all affect how successful an ECV procedure is. The ECV success rate typically falls between 40% and 60%. The success rate is often greater for women who have already given birth, typically ranging from 60% to 70%.

Risks

Although ECV is usually regarded as safe, there are several hazards associated with it, such as:

- **Fetal Distress**: If the baby becomes distressed during the process, it may need an emergency cesarean section or other urgent medical attention.

- **Preterm Labor:** Sometimes uterine manipulation results in preterm labor.

- **Placental Abruption:** This might cause serious difficulties if the placenta partly separates from the uterine wall.

- **Uterine Rupture:** Although incredibly rare, uterine rupture is a possibility, particularly in women whose uteruses have scars from prior surgery.

Preparation and Expectations

Before the Procedure

- **Pre-Procedure advice**: Before the procedure, the healthcare practitioner will provide detailed advice on what to eat, and drink, and how to take medications.

- **Support Person:** If you need emotional support or help getting home, it's a good idea to bring along a support person.

During the Process:

- **Pain and Discomfort**: During ECV, some pain and discomfort are typical. Although each woman experiences discomfort differently, the process shouldn't be unduly uncomfortable.

- **Communication**: The mother should notify the healthcare practitioner right away if she experiences any acute pain or discomfort.

After the Procedure:

- **Observation**: To make sure there are no urgent difficulties, the woman will be observed for a while.

- **Follow-Up**: If the ECV is not successful, a follow-up session is often arranged to verify the baby's position and go over the next actions.

Chiropractic Techniques (Webster Technique)

A chiropractic technique called the Webster Technique focuses on pelvic alignment and releases tension in the uterine ligaments to treat breech presentation. The goal of this method is to improve the environment so that the infant can naturally flip head-down.

How It Works

Pelvic Alignment

To lessen misalignments and enhance general pelvic balance, the Webster Technique includes precise chiropractic adjustments to the pelvis. A well-aligned pelvis can release restrictions that can keep the baby from rotating and increase the amount of room inside the uterus.

Uterine Ligament Tension

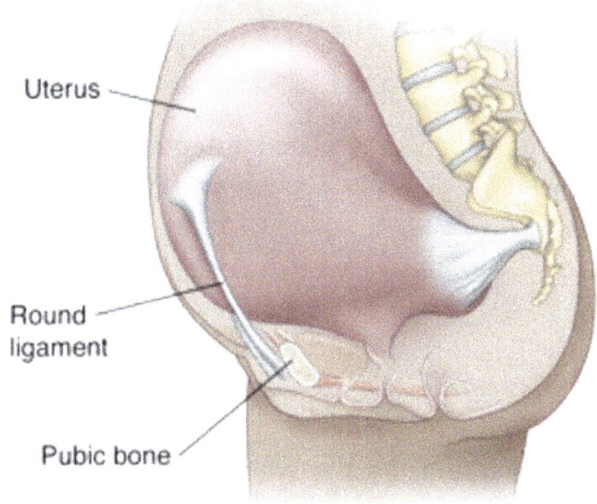

The method also takes care of the circular ligaments that support the uterus. The uterus can take on a more ideal shape and position, allowing the baby to move more easily, by releasing tension in these ligaments.

Locating a Qualified Practitioner Certification and Training

Specific training and certification are required for chiropractors who use the Webster Technique. Chiropractors can get certified in this approach by joining the International Chiropractic Pediatric Association (ICPA).

Selecting a Chiropractor:

- **Experience**: Seek a chiropractor who has used the Webster Technique and knows prenatal care.

- **Referrals and Reviews:** To locate a trustworthy practitioner, ask friends, family, or medical professionals for referrals. You may also check internet reviews.

- **Consultation**: Make an appointment for a consultation to go over the chiropractor's method and make sure you're comfortable receiving their care.

Research and Effectiveness

Research and Results

There is little, but encouraging, research on the Webster Technique's efficacy. When a trained professional uses this approach to turn a breech baby, some studies indicate a success rate of about 70%. More thorough scientific research is needed to validate these results, though.

Experiences of Patients

In addition to noting increased comfort and decreased pregnancy-related discomforts, many women report excellent results and great satisfaction with the Webster Technique. It also can flip a breech baby.

Safety Points to Remember

- **Non-Invasive:** When carried out by a qualified chiropractor, the Webster Technique is a minimally invasive technique with little danger. Since it doesn't need any medicine or surgery, many expectant mothers find it to be a safe alternative.

- **Restrictions**: Before receiving chiropractic therapy, women with certain medical issues or complications—such as placenta previa or a high-risk pregnancy—should speak with their healthcare physician.

Moxibustion and Acupuncture

Chinese traditional medicine has long employed moxibustion and acupuncture to treat a variety of ailments, including breech presentation. These techniques entail applying pressure to particular body areas to induce the infant to flip to facedown.

Methods of Traditional Chinese Medicine

- **Acupuncture**: Fine needles are inserted into certain body spots, or acupoints, during an acupuncture session. The main acupoint for breech presentation is BL-67, which is situated close to the pinky toe's outer corner. It is thought that stimulating this site would encourage fetal movement and uterine contractions.

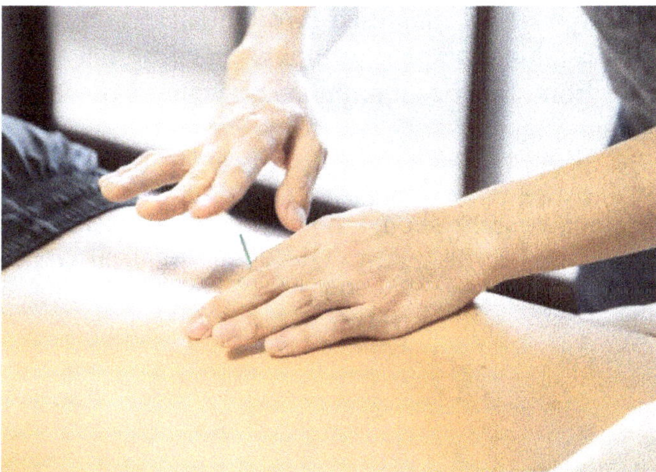

- **Moxibustion**: To create heat and activate certain acupoints, mugwort (Artemisia vulgaris) is burned close to the points. To maximize the benefits of acupuncture, this technique is frequently combined with it. Moxibustion is usually given to the BL-67 point for breech presentation.

Research and Effectiveness

- **Clinical research:** Several clinical research have looked at the efficacy of moxibustion and acupuncture in turning breech newborns. When compared to no intervention, a meta-analysis of randomized controlled studies indicates that these methods can raise the chance of the baby going head-down. Studies have shown varying success rates, although they typically fall between 30% and 70%.

- **Processes of Action:** There is still some confusion regarding the precise processes via which moxibustion and acupuncture operate. Nonetheless, it's thought that activating particular acupoints might boost fetal movement and improve the environment in which the baby turns.

Safety Points to Remember

- **Professionals with the necessary qualifications**: Seeking care from a licensed and skilled acupuncturist who is knowledgeable about prenatal care and the particular methods for turning a breech baby is imperative.

- **Safety Profile:** When administered by a qualified professional, moxibustion and acupuncture are usually regarded as safe therapies. Although they are uncommon, side effects might include slight burns from moxibustion, minor bruising, and soreness at the locations where needles are inserted.

- **Precautions**: Acupuncture and moxibustion should not be used in cases of placenta previa, premature labor, or certain medical disorders. Always get medical advice before beginning any of these procedures.

CHAPTER FIVE

Alternative and Holistic Methods (Intermediate Level)

While non-medical procedures and conventional medical measures can frequently assist in turning a breech baby, some parents may choose to use holistic and alternative approaches. These methods incorporate mental and emotional health in addition to physical treatments, and they frequently offer a more thorough and non-intrusive strategy to urge the baby to turn its head down.

This chapter explores several complementary and alternative techniques, including visualization, hypnobirthing, talking to the baby, and using heat and cold. Comprehensive explanations, step-by-step instructions, success stories, and safety concerns will all be included in each part.

Hypnobirthing and Visualization

Understanding Hypnobirthing

Hypnobirthing is a method that encourages a peaceful and optimistic attitude throughout pregnancy and labor by employing self-hypnosis, relaxation, and visualization. The basic idea is that although relaxation and positive imagery might promote a more painless birthing experience, fear and tension can cause pain and difficulties.

Although hypnobirthing is frequently connected to labor, it can also be used to turn a breech baby.

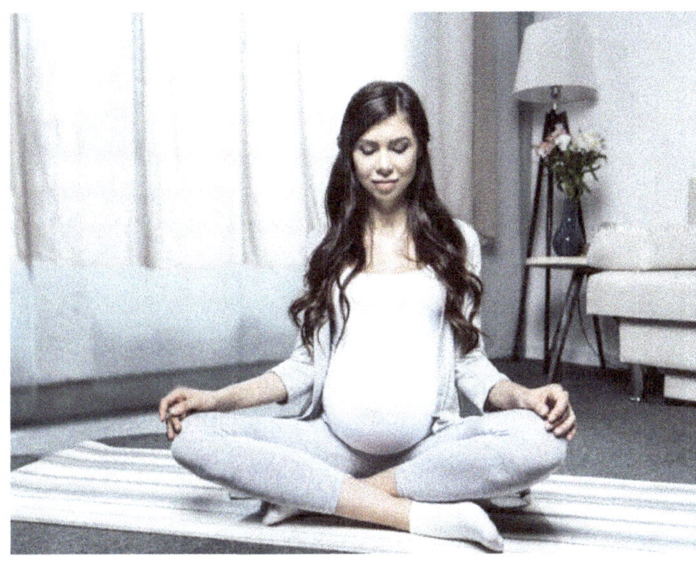

Methods and Approaches

Affirmations, deep breathing exercises, and guided visualizations are some of the hypnobirthing methods used to turn a breech baby.

Here is a thorough how-to:

1. **Guided Visualizations:**

- **Visualization**: Imagine the fetus tilting its head down in the womb. Imagine the infant settling into the proper posture with ease and gentleness.

- **Setting the Scene**: Make sure everything is quiet and uncluttered. To improve relaxation, use soft lighting, relaxing music, or sounds of the natural world.

- **Consistency**: Use these visualizations regularly, preferably in a calm and cozy environment.

2. **Deep Relaxation Exercises:**

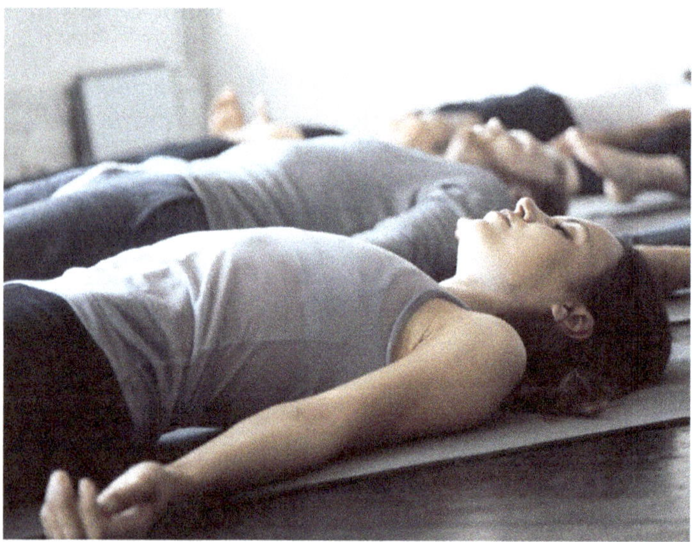

- **Progressive Muscle Relaxation**: Work your way up to the head by gradually tensing and relaxing various muscle groups, beginning with the feet. This encourages general relaxation and relieves physical strain.

- **Breathing exercises:** Pay attention to calm, deep breaths. Breathe in from your nose, hold it for a short while, and then gently release the air through your mouth. This promotes increased oxygen flow and calms the neurological system.

3. **Affirmations:**

- **Positive Statements**: Repeat positive statements every day to help you maintain a good outlook. Some examples of these affirmations are "**My baby is turning head-down" and "I am relaxed and my baby is moving into the correct position.**"

Success Stories

The usefulness of hypnobirthing and visualization in flipping breech infants is demonstrated by several success stories. For example, Californian mother Sarah talked about how she turned her 36-week-old breech baby around with the help of affirmations and guided visualizations. She credits the turn's success to the regular use of these strategies together with a serene and upbeat outlook.

Safety Points to Remember

For the majority of pregnant women, hypnobirthing and visualization are typically safe.

Still, it's critical to:

- **Speak with a Healthcare Professional:** Make sure the methods are suitable for your particular circumstance by discussing them with your midwife or obstetrician.

- **Prevent Overexertion:** Make sure you execute relaxation techniques in a strain-free and comfortable manner.

Talking to Your Baby

Communicating with Your Baby in the Womb

Talking to your unborn child can help you build a close emotional bond with them and may even urge them to turn over onto their head. Using touch, talking to your kid, and playing music are all part of this strategy.

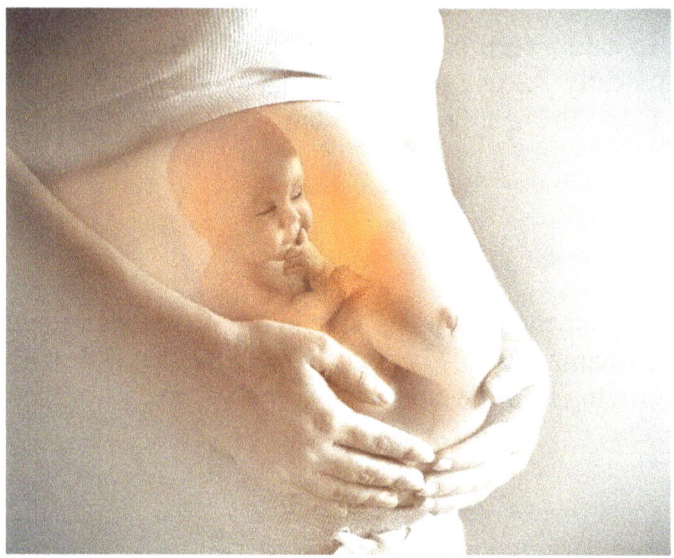

Techniques for Communicating

1. **Speaking to Your Baby**:

- **Calm and Reassuring Voice**: Use a soothing, tranquil voice when speaking to your infant. In plain, loving words, tell them you want them to turn heads down.

- **Regular Conversations**: Include these talks in your everyday schedule, for example, before bed or in the morning.

2. **Using Touch**

- **Belly massage:** Gently rub your stomach, paying particular attention to the spots where the baby moves. To provide a soothing experience, move in circular motions and apply gentle pressure.

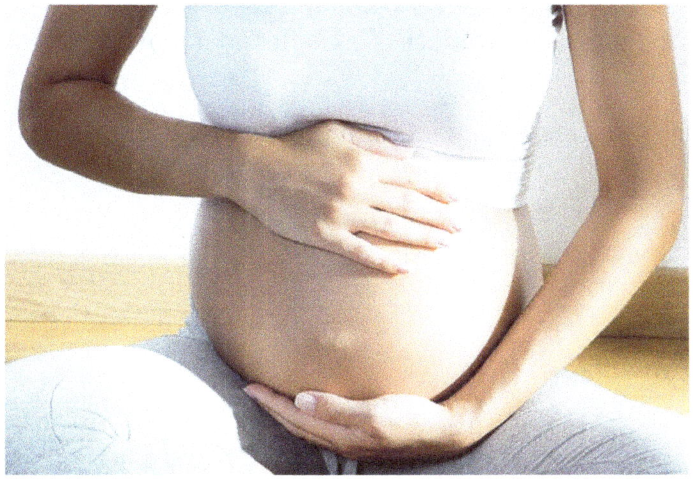

- **Tummy Mapping**: Use touch to try to determine your baby's location. This will assist you in determining where to concentrate your efforts.

3. **Playing Music:**

- **Lower Belly Placement:** Play soothing music using headphones or a speaker next to your lower abdomen. Because they are drawn to noises, babies may gravitate toward music.

- **Consistent Timing**: To promote exercise, play music at regular intervals throughout the day.

Success Stories

Many parents have reported success stories when they used communication to help their breech babies turn. Maria is one such tale; she talked to her infant all the time and had classical music playing close to her belly. Her baby turned head-down at 37 weeks, which she credits to the supportive and peaceful atmosphere she fostered.

Safety Points to Remember

It's safe and beneficial for mother and child to communicate with each other about their needs and wants.

Think about the following:

- **Gentle Touch**: Be sure that any massages or touches are soft and not overly strong.

- **Volume Control**: To prevent shocking the infant, turn down the music to a comfortable level.

Applying Cold and Heat

The Concept of Heat and Cold Application

The idea behind applying heat and cold is that infants tend to gravitate toward warmth and away from cold. Head-down can be encouraged by parents delivering cold or heat strategically to certain parts of the abdomen.

Techniques for Applying Heat and Cold

1. **Heat Application:**

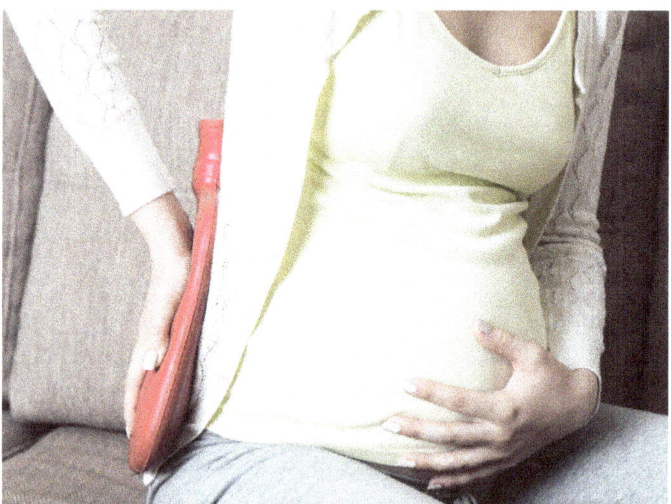

- **Warm Compress:** Apply a low-temperature heating pad or warm compress to the lower region of your abdomen. The infant may approach it because of its warmth.

- **Warm Baths:** Giving your infant a warm bath might help them to reposition themselves and provide a soothing atmosphere.

2. **Cold Application:**

- **Cold Compress**: Apply a cold compress or a cloth-wrapped bag of frozen peas to the top region of your belly. The infant can be encouraged to move away from it by the chilly feeling.

- **Rotating Heat and Cold**: For ten minutes at a time, switch between heating the lower abdomen and cooling the upper belly.

Success Stories

For some parents, the use of heat and cold has proven beneficial. For instance, Jessica, a mother from New York, turned her breech baby at 35 weeks of pregnancy by using a mix of warm baths and cold compresses. She discovered that this approach worked well for getting her baby to move when paired with relaxing techniques.

Safety Points to Remember

When done properly, applying heat and cold is typically safe. Observe these rules:

- **Temperature Control**: To prevent pain or damage, make sure the compresses are not excessively hot or too cold.

- **Time Limits:** To avoid irritating skin, apply heat or cold for no more than ten to fifteen minutes at a time.

Combining Techniques for Optimal Results

Creating a Holistic Approach

A synergistic effect can be produced by combining several holistic and alternative approaches, which increases the chance of turning a breech baby. Through the integration of hypnobirthing, temperature approaches, and communication, parents may create a customized and all-encompassing strategy.

Customized Schedule

1. **Daily Schedule:**
- **Morning**: In the morning, take a warm bath after doing a guided visualization and affirmations.

- **Afternoon**: In the afternoon, play relaxing music and give yourself a belly rub.

- **Evening**: At night, talk to your child in a calming tone and use hot and cold compresses.

2. **Continuity and Flexibility:**

- **Consistent Practice**: Make sure you practice these methods daily.

- **Flexibility**: Modify the regimen following comfort and efficacy, seeking advice from a healthcare professional as necessary.

Success Stories

Parents who have integrated approaches effectively tend to report greater success rates. For example, Emily, a Texas woman, combined hypnobirthing with talking to her infant and using heat and cold. Her baby went head-down at 36 weeks, and she credits her comprehensive, methodical approach for the success of this birth.

Safety Pointers

When mixing methods, it's critical to:

- **Keep an eye on Comfort:** Make sure that no practice is stressful or uncomfortable.

- **Consult Healthcare Providers**: To ensure safety and appropriateness, regularly review your strategy with your healthcare practitioner.

Integrating Partner Support

The Role of Partners

Partners may be very important in helping the mother and making these holistic approaches successful. Their participation may foster a supportive and upbeat atmosphere, assist with practical procedures, and offer emotional support.

Techniques for Partner Involvement

1. **Participation in Hypnobirthing**:

- **Guided Sessions:** Spoken direction and support can be given by partners during hypnobirthing sessions.

- **Affirmations**: To help the mother maintain a good outlook, partners might repeat affirmations to her.

2. **Support for Communication:**

- **Talking to the Baby:** By engaging in dialogue with the infant, partners can foster a feeling of togetherness and purpose.

- **Playing Music**: To ensure that the music is relaxing and enjoyable, partners can assist in selecting and playing it.

3. **Using Cold and Heat:**

- **Heat Compress**: Partners can help ensure that heat compresses are used and prepared at a suitable degree.

- **Cold Compress:** Partners can assist in applying cold compresses while keeping an eye on the patient's comfort level and time.

Success Stories

The efficiency of these methods can be increased when partners are involved. The story of Laura and James, who collaborated through temperature, communication, and hypnobirthing methods, serves as one example. At 37 weeks, their breech baby turned head-down as a consequence of their combined efforts.

Safety Points to Remember

When collaborating with others, it's critical to:

- **Be Open with Communication:** Make sure that both partners feel at ease and are aware of the strategies being used.

- **Function as a Team**: Be patient, cooperative, and adaptable as you go through the process.

Professional Support for Alternative Methods

Seeking Professional Guidance

While many holistic and alternative techniques may be used at home, getting expert advice can increase their efficacy and guarantee safety. Experts like acupuncturists, chiropractors, and hypnobirthing teachers can offer customized guidance and specialized assistance.

Hypnobirthing Instructors

1. **Locating a Reputable Teacher:**

- **Credentials**: Seek for hypnobirthing teachers who have received certification and have worked with breech pregnancies.

- **Referrals**: Ask other parents or medical professionals for suggestions.

2. **What to anticipate:**

- **Sessions**: Teachers usually provide one-on-one or group instruction in affirmations, visualizations, and relaxation methods.

- **Resources**: Instructors could offer extra materials like guided visualization recordings and relaxation techniques.

Chiropractors and the Webster Technique

1. **Understanding the Webster Technique:**

- **Goal**: To provide the best possible environment for the baby to turn, the Webster Technique focuses on pelvic alignment and uterine tension reduction.

- **Technique**: A chiropractor will employ mild adjustments to the surrounding muscles and pelvis.

2. **Locating a Skilled Chiropractor:**

- **Credentials**: Seek chiropractors with experience in prenatal treatment and certification in the Webster Technique.

- **Recommendations**: See your midwife or obstetrician for suggestions.

Moxibustion and Acupuncturists

1. **Understanding Moxibustion and Acupuncture:**

- **Acupuncture**: This modality of healing involves stimulating movement by putting tiny needles into particular body locations.

- **Moxibustion**: This technique involves lighting a herb close to designated spots to provide warmth and entice the infant to turn.

2. **Locating an Accredited Acupuncturist:**

- **Credentials**: Seek acupuncturists who are licensed and have treated breech pregnancies before.

- **Referrals**: Ask for advice from medical professionals or other reliable sources.

Success Stories

Expert assistance can greatly improve the efficacy of alternative approaches. For instance, Samantha, a Florida woman, successfully turned her 36-week-old breech baby by working with a chiropractor and hypnobirthing teacher. She discovered that the combination of at-home methods and expert advice worked well.

Safety Points to Remember

When pursuing expert assistance, it's crucial to:

- **Check Credentials:** Make sure experts have the necessary training and experience in their domains.

- **Communicate Openly:** To guarantee comfort and clarity, discuss any worries or inquiries with the experts.

Monitoring Progress and Adjusting Techniques

Tracking Baby's Position

It is essential to often observe the baby's posture to evaluate the efficacy of the procedures and make any required modifications. Ultrasounds, self-monitoring, and prenatal checkups can all help with this.

Techniques for Self-Monitoring

1. **Tummy Mapping:**

- **Identify Movements**: Observe the baby's movements and make an effort to chart their location by feeling various areas of the abdomen.

- **Use a Guide**: To precisely determine the baby's position, use a belly mapping guide or consult a doula or midwife.

2. **Kick Counts:**

- **Track Movement:** Count the baby's motions regularly to keep an eye on their position and level of activity. An active baby is more likely to turn.

Adjusting Techniques

Parents may need to modify their strategies to increase efficacy in light of the monitoring outcomes.

Here's how to do it:

1. **If There Is No Progress:**

- **Change Routine**: Modify the methods' frequency and timing. For instance, extend the time spent doing relaxation techniques or alternate between applying heat and cold.

- **Consult Experts:** Get more advice from medical professionals or experts such as chiropractors or hypnobirthing teachers.

2. **If Baby Starts to Turn:**

- **Continue Techniques**: To motivate the infant to finish their turn, stick to the present schedule.

- **Increase Frequency**: To reinforce the beneficial changes, increase the frequency of effective procedures.

Success Stories

Parents who keep a close eye on things and make necessary adjustments frequently report positive results. For example, Amanda, a mother from Colorado, tracked her baby's whereabouts using kick counts and stomach mapping. She flipped her breech baby at 35 weeks by modifying her regimen according to the baby's motions.

Safety Points to Remember

When evaluating and modifying methods, take into account the following:

- **Prevent Overexertion:** Make sure that any modifications are done in a relaxed and painless manner.

- **Consult Healthcare Providers:** To ensure safety and appropriateness, discuss any changes with your healthcare provider regularly.

Mental and Emotional Health

The Value of Mental Well-Being

Pregnancy requires maintaining one's emotional and mental well, particularly while handling a breech presentation. Anxiety and stress can affect both the overall pregnancy experience and the efficacy of the procedures.

Methods for Improving Wellness

1. **Meditation & Mindfulness:**
- **Mindfulness Techniques**: To stay present and lower anxiety, practice mindfulness. This might involve mindful walking or basic breathing techniques.

- **Meditation**: To encourage calmness and an optimistic outlook, use guided meditations created especially for expectant mothers.

2. **Support Systems:**

- **Friends and Family**: Seek out emotional support from friends and family. Talk to them about your worries and experiences.

- **Support Groups**: Participate in groups designed to assist expectant mothers or those facing breech deliveries. Sharing with others might bring solace and insightful perspectives.

3. **Therapeutic Approaches:**

- **Counseling**: Take into consideration consulting with a therapist or counselor who specializes in prenatal care. They can offer emotional support and coping mechanisms.

- **Journaling**: Write down your ideas and emotions in a notebook. This can lessen tension and aid in the processing of emotions.

Success Stories

Positive results might arise from concentrating on one's emotional and mental health. For instance, Oregonian mother Claire utilized mindfulness and meditation to control her worry over her breech baby. At 34 weeks, she discovered that keeping her mind at ease and thinking positively assisted her baby's turn.

Safety Points to Remember

When concentrating on one's mental and emotional health, it is crucial to:

- **Seek Professional Assistance:** Consult a counselor or therapist if you're suffering from severe depression or anxiety.

- **Balance Techniques:** To preserve general wellbeing, make sure that relaxation methods are balanced with other everyday activities.

CHAPTER SIX

Problem-Solving and Troubleshooting

For pregnant parents, seeing a breech presentation throughout the prenatal journey might be frightening. But knowing what methods and procedures are available to turn a breech baby is just one step in the process.

This chapter concentrates on problem-solving and troubleshooting, including comprehensive instructions on what to do if these methods prove ineffective, controlling tension and anxiety, and comprehending medical advice.

When Techniques Don't Work

Sometimes the ways to turn a breech baby won't work, even with the greatest of intentions. This section delves into the causes of method failures and provides an outline of future actions and alternate approaches.

Understanding the Reasons Behind Technique Failure

When trying to flip a breech infant, there are a few things that might go wrong:

- **Gestational Age**: As pregnancy goes on, the uterus's volume narrows and the baby finds it more difficult to turn.

- **Uterine Abnormalities**: The baby's range of motion may be restricted by structural problems such as fibroids or a bicornuate uterus.

- **Placental Position**: A low-lying placenta, such as placenta previa, might physically prevent the infant from rotating.

- **Amniotic Fluid Levels**: A baby's ability to move may be impacted by oligohydramnios, little amniotic fluid, polyhydramnios, or excess amniotic fluid.

- **Baby's Size and Position**: It might be more difficult for larger newborns or those in a highly flexed position to turn.

By being aware of these variables, parents and healthcare professionals may make appropriate adjustments to their approach and ascertain why some strategies might not be effective.

Re-evaluating Techniques

If the baby refuses to turn, it's critical to reassess the methods used:

- **Frequency and Duration**: You may get better benefits by doing exercises like pelvic tilts and forward-leaning inversions more frequently or for longer periods.

- **Combination of Techniques:** Combining techniques can increase efficacy. For example, mother positioning exercises can be used in addition to chiropractic therapy.

- **Professional Guidance:** Consulting with medical professionals, such as chiropractors, obstetricians, or midwives, might yield new perspectives and methods that were previously unconsidered.

Subsequent Actions and Other Plans

Other approaches that can be investigated in case of failure of traditional procedures include:

- **External Cephalic Version (ECV):** A qualified obstetrician will manually turn the baby from the outside by pressing on the abdomen during this technique. ECV contains considerable hazards and may not be appropriate for all pregnancies, despite its remarkable success rate.

- **Scheduled Cesarean Section:** This may be the safest course of action if the infant stays breech. Complications from vaginal breech birth can be avoided with this surgical treatment.

- **Vaginal Breech Delivery:** This option could be taken into consideration in specific circumstances. This calls for a knowledgeable and experienced healthcare professional, and it is usually only advised in certain circumstances where the advantages exceed the disadvantages.

Handling Stress and Anxiety

Being pregnant is an emotional roller coaster, and having a breech presentation may make things even more stressful and anxious. This section provides ways for efficiently coping with certain emotions.

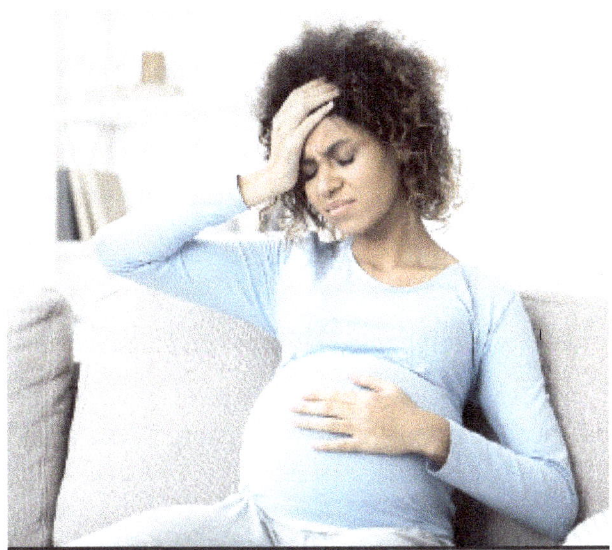

Parental Coping Strategies

Parents must learn coping skills to handle the emotional difficulties brought on by a breech pregnancy:

- **Mindfulness and Meditation**: These two techniques can ease anxiety and encourage calm. Particularly helpful techniques include gradual muscular relaxation, guided visualization, and deep breathing.

- **Support Networks:** Establishing a robust support system with loved ones, close friends, and medical professionals may offer consolation and useful guidance. Parents can connect with others facing similar issues by attending in-person or online support groups.

- **Therapeutic Interventions:** Consulting a mental health expert, such as a therapist or counselor, can offer further assistance. Anxiety and stress can be managed with the use of cognitive-behavioral therapy (CBT) and other therapeutic techniques.

Partner Support

To control the emotional effects of a breech presentation, a partner's involvement is essential:

- **Active Participation**: Partners can offer both physical and emotional assistance by actively engaging in exercises and procedures to turn the infant.

- **Emotional Availability**: Anxiety can be reduced and a sense of shared responsibility can be fostered by being emotionally accessible, listening, and providing reassurance.

- **Attending visits:** Partner education and involvement in decision-making may be maintained by accompanying the expecting mother to doctor's visits.

Lifestyle Adjustments

During this period, modifying some aspects of your lifestyle might also help you manage stress:

- **Healthy Diet**: Eating a nutritious, well-balanced diet can help with energy levels and general well-being.

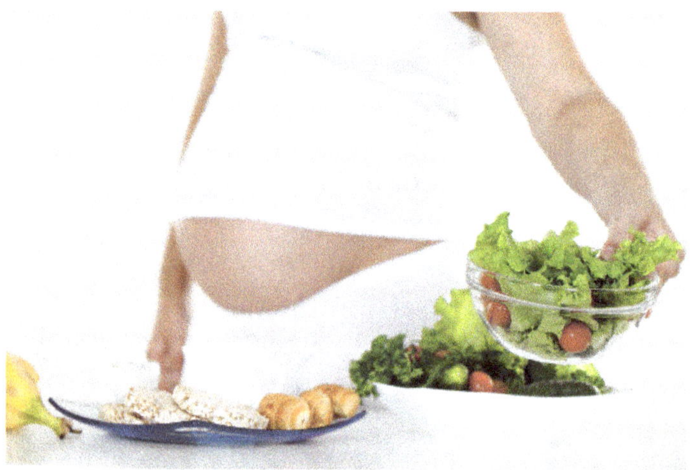

- **Frequent Exercise:** Walking or prenatal yoga are two examples of regular, mild exercise that can enhance mood and physical well-being.

- **Sufficient Rest:** Stress management and preserving physical health depend on getting enough sleep and rest.

Understanding Medical Advice

It might be difficult to navigate medical guidance, particularly in the case of a breech presentation. The purpose of this part is to make sure parents are informed and to demystify medical advice.

Interpreting Monitoring and Ultrasound Data

To evaluate the position and general health of the baby, routine ultrasounds and monitoring are essential. Making sense of these findings is crucial to decision-making:

- **Results from Ultrasounds**: Ultrasounds can give precise views of the placenta's position, amniotic fluid levels, and baby's position. The ramifications of these results can be explained by healthcare practitioners.

- **Non-Stress Tests (NST):** NSTs track the heart rate and movements of the infant. Parents may keep updated on their baby's health by being aware of how these tests are carried out and what the results mean.

- **Doppler studies:** These investigations gauge blood flow across various arteries, including the umbilical artery. These investigations can shed light on the placenta's role and the health of the fetus.

Knowing When to Consider Cesarean

When a baby is a breech, sometimes the safest course of action is a cesarean section.

Knowing when to make this choice can help parents become ready:

- **Medical Indications**: Depending on the mother's health and pregnancy history, as well as the baby's size, position, and general health, medical professionals may advise a cesarean section.

- **Emergencies**: An early cesarean section may be required in some emergency conditions, such as umbilical cord prolapse or fetal distress.

- **Making Informed Decisions**: Talking with medical professionals about the advantages and disadvantages of a cesarean section can assist parents in making well-informed decisions and getting ready, both physically and psychologically, for the operation.

Recognizing the Benefits and Risks

Every intervention has advantages and disadvantages, whether it is medical or not. Parents who are aware of these can make well-rounded decisions:

- **Medical Risks:** Risks associated with medical procedures like epidural catheterization (ECV) and cesarean sections include infection, hemorrhage, and anesthesia-related side effects. Providers of healthcare can go into great depth about these hazards.

- **Non-Medical Risks**: If not used properly, non-medical methods like specific workouts or alternative therapies can potentially be dangerous. It's critical to heed advice and suggestions from professionals.

- **Balancing Benefits**: Parents can select the best course of action for their unique scenario by weighing the advantages of each intervention against any potential hazards.

When Techniques Don't Work

It might be depressing to come across a breech presentation that doesn't improve with repeated therapies. Effectively handling this scenario requires recognizing why these strategies might not work as well as knowing what to do next.

Understanding the Reasons Behind Technique Failure

Techniques to turn a breech infant may fail for several reasons. These can be generally divided into environmental, mother-related, and baby-related variables.

Maternal Factors

- **Uterine Anomalies:** An infant's range of motion may be restricted by structural uterine abnormalities, such as fibroids or a bicornuate uterus.

- **Pelvic Shape**: Certain women have a pelvic shape that hinders the baby's ability to spin.

- **Amniotic Fluid Levels:** A baby's ability to move may be impacted by oligohydramnios, little amniotic fluid, polyhydramnios, or excess amniotic fluid. Movement is restricted by low fluid, and maintaining a head-down position might be challenging due to abundant fluid.

Fetal Factors

- **Size and Gestational Age**: Babies who are larger or near term have less space to maneuver, which makes turning more difficult.

- **Position and Engagement:** Turning a baby is more difficult if its head is already positioned breech inside the pelvis.

- **Cord Position:** An infant may occasionally be unable to turn safely due to the position of the umbilical cord.

Environmental Factors

- **Timing and Consistency**: Two important factors are timing and consistency while using approaches. Exercises done inconsistently or too late in the pregnancy, for instance, would not be beneficial.

- **Maternal Activity Levels:** Certain strategies may be less successful in a sedentary lifestyle. Frequent, mild exercise can help the infant move.

Re-evaluating Techniques

If the baby won't flip over after trying a few times, it's crucial to review the techniques and think of other options.

- **The Duration and Frequency**

It may be possible to increase the efficacy of some workouts by increasing their frequency and duration. To get the baby to turn, for instance, pelvic tilts and forward-leaning inversions may need to be done more often or held for longer periods.

- **Combination of Techniques**

Combining several approaches can increase their overall efficacy. For example, employing acupuncture or chiropractic treatments in addition to maternal positioning exercises may yield greater benefits than using either technique alone.

- **Professional Guidance**

Consulting with medical professionals who specialize in breech presentations might yield fresh perspectives and methods. Chiropractors, acupuncturists, midwives, and obstetricians may all provide individualized advice and assistance.

Next Steps and Alternative Strategies

If traditional methods are ineffective, investigating substitute approaches and becoming ready for possible results becomes crucial.

External Cephalic Version (ECV)

An experienced obstetrician can manually turn the baby from the outside using an ECV method. Usually, it is done between weeks 36 and 37 of pregnancy. ECV has a 50–60% success rate and is regarded as quite safe when carried out by qualified professionals. Nonetheless, there are a few hazards, such as:

- **Fetal Distress:** An emergency cesarean section may be necessary if the surgery results in fetal distress.

- **Premature Rupture of Membranes:** Premature rupture of the membranes can be caused by uterine manipulation, and this can start labor.

- **Placental Abruption**: While uncommon, placental abruption can occur during the surgery.

To make an educated choice about using ECV, parents should talk to their healthcare professional about the advantages and disadvantages of this technology.

Planned Cesarean Delivery

A planned cesarean section may be the safest course of action if the baby stays breech. This makes it possible for medical professionals to organize and be ready for the birth, guaranteeing the best possible outcome for the mother and child. A planned cesarean section should take the following factors into account:

- **Timing**: To balance the advantages of full-term development with the hazards of spontaneous labor, cesarean procedures are often scheduled at 39 weeks or so.

- **Preparation**: Parents should talk to their healthcare practitioner about the specifics of the surgery, the healing process, and any potential issues.

Vaginal Breech Delivery

A vaginal breech birth might be an option in some circumstances. This calls for a highly qualified and experienced healthcare professional, and it is usually only advised in certain circumstances where the advantages exceed the disadvantages.

Considerations for a vaginal breech birth consist of the following:

- **Breech Type:** Compared to a footling breech, frank breech is a more advantageous breech posture for vaginal delivery.

- **Fetal and Maternal Health:** For a vaginal birth to be performed, the mother and child must be in excellent health.

- **Hospital Resources:** If an emergency cesarean section is required, the birth should happen at a hospital with the requisite equipment.

Managing Stress and Anxiety

For pregnant parents, handling a breech presentation can be nerve-wracking and distressing. To maintain a healthy pregnancy, this section focuses on practical ways to handle these emotions.

Meditation and Mindfulness

Meditation and mindfulness techniques may greatly lower anxiety and increase calm. Methods that assist soothe the body and mind include gradual muscle relaxation, guided meditation, and deep breathing.

- **Deep Breathing:** Taking slow, deep breaths helps lower tension and trigger the body's relaxation response.

- **Guided imagery:** Focusing on a calm setting or a successful result can help divert attention from tension and worry.

- **Progressive Muscle Relaxation:** You may assist relieve physical stress and encourage relaxation by tensing and then relaxing various muscle groups.

Support Networks

Creating a solid support system of friends, family, and medical professionals may help with both practical guidance and emotional support.

- **Friends and Family:** Seeking assistance from close ones may be consoling and reassuring.

- **Support Groups**: Parents can meet others going through comparable struggles by joining support groups, either locally or virtually. The exchange of insights and counsel might prove to be immensely advantageous.

Therapeutic Interventions

Consulting a mental health expert, such as a therapist or counselor, might offer further assistance. Anxiety and stress can be managed with the use of cognitive-behavioral therapy (CBT) and other therapeutic techniques.

- **Cognitive-Behavioral Therapy (CBT):** CBT can assist in reframing unfavorable ideas and creating coping mechanisms.

- **Therapy Sessions:** Attending therapy sessions regularly might offer a secure setting for discussing worries and getting expert advice.

Partner Support

To control the emotional effects of a breech presentation, a partner's participation is essential. Partners can provide emotional and physical assistance.

Active Involvement

To turn the infant, partners can actively engage in activities and strategies that offer both physical and emotional assistance.

- **Exercise Participation**: Engaging in exercises like forward-leaning inversions and pelvic tilts can boost confidence and foster a sense of teamwork.

- **Collaborating on Research**: Collaborating on research projects and investigating various methods and strategies can support well-informed decision-making.

Emotional Availability

In addition to reducing fear, providing reassurance and being emotionally present may also promote a sense of shared responsibility.

- **Honesty in Communication**: Keeping lines of communication open and honest about worries and fears helps improve the relationship.

- **Support and Reassurance**: Providing consolation in the form of words and tangible comfort can assist lessen anxiety.

Attending Appointments

Partners who accompany their pregnant spouse to doctor's appointments can remain informed and involved in the decision-making process.

- **Medical Appointments:** Partners can better comprehend the situation and participate in conversations with healthcare providers by attending pregnancy check-ups and consultations.

- **Ultrasound Visits**: Being there during an ultrasound can assist partners stay involved in the procedure and view the baby's location.

Lifestyle Adjustments

During this period, modifying some aspects of your lifestyle might also aid in stress management.

Healthy Diet

Sustaining a nutrient-dense, well-balanced diet can improve energy levels and general well-being. Consuming an array of fruits, vegetables, complete grains, and lean meats can supply the nutrients required for a successful pregnancy.

- **Nutrient-rich foods:** Eating foods high in vitamins and minerals, such as fish, almonds, and leafy greens, can improve both physical and mental well-being.

- **Hydration**: Drinking lots of water will help you stay hydrated, which can lower your stress level and preserve your energy.

Regular Exercise

Regularly doing mild exercise, like walking or yoga for pregnant women, can enhance both mental and physical well-being. Endorphins are released during exercise and have the potential to lower stress and enhance general well-being.

- **Prenatal yoga:** Yoga helps increase strength, relaxation, and flexibility. Stress-reduction breathing techniques are also included.

- **Walking**: Taking regular walks might improve mood by offering mild exercise and a chance to spend time outside.

Adequate Rest

Getting enough sleep and rest is crucial for stress management and preserving physical health. Enhancing sleep quality may be achieved by maintaining a regular sleep schedule and creating a pleasant sleeping environment.

- **Sleep Routine:** Establishing a consistent bedtime and wake-up time each day might assist control sleep habits.

- **Comfortable Environment**: Better sleep may be achieved by creating a peaceful, distraction-free sleeping environment.

CHAPTER SEVEN

Special Cases and Considerations (Senior Level)

The intricacies and subtleties of handling breech presentation in unique situations are covered in detail in Chapter 7. Certain situations call for further considerations and customized methods, even though the broad tactics and interventions covered in previous chapters can be successful in certain cases. Three major topics are covered in this chapter: numerous pregnancies, prior breech deliveries, and high-risk pregnancies. Parents and healthcare professionals may handle these exceptional situations with more assurance and effectiveness if they comprehend the particular difficulties and provide thoughtful solutions.

Multiple Pregnancies

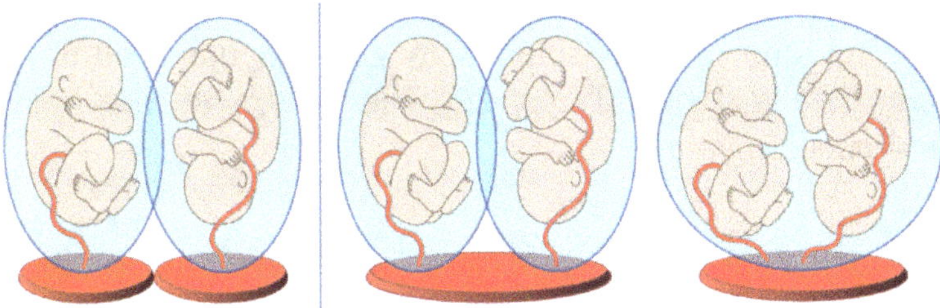

Twins, triplets, and higher-order multiple pregnancies pose special difficulties for parents and medical professionals. The placement, movement, and birth of multiple fetuses can be greatly impacted by their existence in the uterus.

Challenges with Twins and More

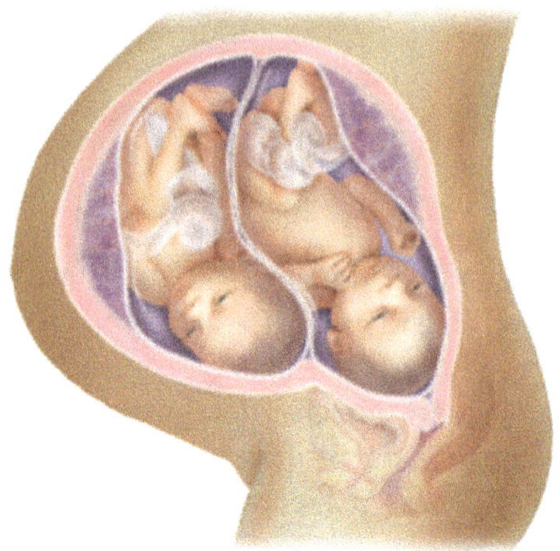

These challenges include the following:

- **Space Restrictions:** The uterus's limited capacity to accommodate numerous pregnancies presents the most evident barrier. Less space for movement exists as fetuses expand, which may make it challenging for one or more infants to get into the head-down position. Due to the limited room, twins frequently appear differently, with one being head-down (vertex) and the other remaining breech.

- **Individual Fetal Movement:** The posture and movement of each baby in a multiple pregnancy might be impacted by the positions of their siblings. For example, a head-down twin may unintentionally limit the mobility of a breech twin, making attempts to turn the latter more difficult.

- **Placental location:** Fetal movement may also be impacted by the placenta's location. A breech infant might be more difficult to flip if the placentas are anterior (front-facing) or positioned in a way that limits room.

- **Amniotic Fluid Levels:** Variations in the amounts of amniotic fluid in twins may affect their motility. There's a chance that one twin has more fluid, which allows for more motion, while the other has less, which restricts movement.

Specific Techniques for Multiples

- **Individualized Assessment:** The location and turning potential of each fetus should be evaluated separately. This involves thorough ultrasonography assessments to comprehend their placement and the amount of room for mobility.

- **Combination approaches**: Due to the intricacies, a mix of medical interventions (like ECV) and non-medical approaches (such as maternal positioning exercises) may be required. To prevent difficulties, these methods must be well coordinated.

- **Simultaneous Monitoring:** To guarantee the safety of every baby during any intervention, it is essential to continuously monitor both fetal heart rates. This may include the deployment of sophisticated monitoring devices that track many heart rhythms at once.

- **Phased birth Planning:** Medical professionals may decide to go forward with a phased birth when dealing with twins that are head-down and breech. This entails vaginally delivering the head-down twin first, then determining the second twin's position. A breech vaginal birth or an emergency cesarean surgery may be considered if the second twin stays breech.

Delivery-Related Issues

- **Cesarean Section:** A scheduled cesarean section is frequently the safest option for higher-order multiples or when the hazards of vaginal birth are judged to be too severe. This is particularly true if a baby or infants are breech, which is a challenging posture for them.

- **Vaginal birth:** A vaginal birth may be attempted in some circumstances, particularly in situations of twins where the first twin is head-down. After the first twin is born, the position of the second twin will be reevaluated, and the necessary steps will be made to guarantee a safe delivery.

- **Multidisciplinary Approach**: When dealing with multiple pregnancies, an interdisciplinary team of obstetricians, experts in maternal-fetal medicine, anesthesiologists, and neonatal specialists is frequently needed. This guarantees the timely and efficient handling of any possible issues.

Past Cases of Breech Births

In their subsequent pregnancies, parents who have already had a breech delivery may have particular worries and considerations. Effective management requires an understanding of their prior experiences and the integration of that information into present initiatives.

Drawing Lessons from the Past

- **Comprehensive Medical History:** It is imperative to do a thorough analysis of the prior breech delivery. This entails comprehending the causes of the breech presentation, the tried therapies, and the results. It is important to identify and treat specific variables, such as placental problems or anomalies in the uterus.

- **Emotional Impact**: It is important to recognize the significant emotional and psychological effects of a prior breech delivery. Parents could feel more fearful and anxious about the same thing happening again. Counseling and emotional support can lessen these worries and encourage a positive perspective.

Customizing Methods Based on Personal Experience

- **Tailored Approach**: A tailored strategy must be devised, taking into consideration the knowledge acquired from the prior encounter. This might entail the employment of certain non-medical practices that have been helpful in the past, earlier and more regular monitoring, or innovative approaches to issues that have been recognized.

- **Enhanced Monitoring**: To keep a closer eye on the location of the fetus, routine ultrasounds and checkups should be planned. This makes it possible to identify breech presentations early and to intervene quickly.

- **Preventive Measures**: Preventive measures should be implemented if the prior breech presentation was caused by uterine anomalies or other physical causes. To address these concerns, this may involve physical therapy, specific exercises, or medicinal interventions.

Preparing for Different Scenarios

- **Flexible Birth Plan:** It is important to create a flexible birth plan that takes into account various circumstances. This plan should be flexible to accommodate the baby's position closer to the due date, and it should contain preferences for both vaginal and cesarean births.

- **Making Informed Decisions**: Parents need to be aware of the advantages and disadvantages of various delivery methods. This involves being aware of the possibility of a repeat breech presentation and the various management strategies that can be used.

- **Supportive Environment:** Establishing a supportive atmosphere can help parents feel more prepared and less nervous. Examples of such environments include peer support groups, breech delivery-focused birthing programs, and access to skilled healthcare experts.

High-Risk Pregnancies

Specialized treatment and a more careful approach to controlling breech presentation are necessary in high-risk pregnancies. Extra vigilance is required due to factors such as past pregnancy problems, advanced maternal age, and maternal health issues.

Extra Safety Measures and Adjustments

- **Comprehensive Risk Assessment**: To detect potential difficulties, a thorough risk assessment should be carried out early in the pregnancy. This includes assessing any prior pregnancy difficulties as well as maternal health issues including hypertension, diabetes, or heart disease.

- **Specialized Care Team**: The engagement of a maternal-fetal medicine specialist might be beneficial in high-risk pregnancies as they can offer knowledgeable counsel and continuous monitoring.

- **Tailored Monitoring Plan:** To closely monitor the health and location of the fetus, a tailored monitoring plan should be developed. This should include more regular ultrasounds and non-stress testing.

Personalized Approaches for High-Risk Pregnancy

- **Non-Medical Approaches with Caution**: In high-risk pregnancies, non-medical approaches such as maternal positioning exercises can be helpful, but they should be used with caution. To make sure they don't worsen pre-existing problems, the healthcare provider should authorize any workouts or postures.

- **Medical therapies:** With extra caution, medical therapies like electroconvulsive therapy (ECV) may still be explored in high-risk pregnancies. The surgery needs to be carried out in a hospital environment with quick access to emergency care in case it's necessary.

- **Holistic treatments:** Although they should be customized to the unique requirements and constraints of the high-risk pregnancy, holistic treatments like acupuncture, chiropractic adjustments, and hypnobirthing can still be helpful. To securely incorporate these techniques, cooperation with healthcare providers is crucial.

Working Intensively with Medical Professionals

Here's how you can work together with medical professionals:

- **Open Communication**: It's critical to keep lines of communication open and consistent with healthcare providers. It should be acceptable for parents to voice any worries and inquire about their alternatives for pregnancy and delivery.

- **Informed Consent:** It is crucial to make sure that parents are completely aware of the advantages and disadvantages of any suggested interventions and delivery strategies. This calls for in-depth conversations and, if needed, the provision of written material.

- **Emergency readiness**: Comprehensive preparations for emergency readiness should be included in high-risk pregnancies. This includes being aware of potential issues, knowing who to call in an emergency, and having a clear strategy for getting to the hospital.

CHAPTER EIGHT

Post-Turn Care and Follow-Up

Following a successful head-down turn, expectant parents and medical professionals must make sure the baby stays in this ideal position and make the necessary arrangements for labor and delivery.

This chapter explores the many facets of follow-up and post-turn care, such as monitoring, making last-minute arrangements, and taking stock of the trip.

Monitoring After a Successful Turn

Keeping an eye on the baby's position following a successful turn is essential to guarantee a risk-free and seamless birth. It is important to have routine check-ups and ultrasounds performed to ensure the baby stays head-down.

The Importance of Constant Monitoring

- **Preventing Reversion:** The baby may still attempt to turn back to a breech position even after a successful rotation. Ongoing observation aids in the early detection of any such reversal.

- **Early Complications Detection**: By doing routine examinations, medical professionals can identify any possible issues that may develop after the infant turns.

- **Comfort for Parents**: Ongoing observation soothes parents, reducing worry and guaranteeing that they are aware of their infant's whereabouts and condition.

Techniques for Observation

- **Frequent Ultrasound Scans:** The most dependable way to verify the baby's location is via an ultrasound scan. Depending on the particulars of each pregnancy, these scans might be conducted at regular intervals.

- **Physical Examinations:** Medical professionals may also palpate the mother's belly during physical examinations, such as Leopold's maneuvers, to determine the baby's position.

- **Monitoring Fetal Movements:** Parents should be urged to keep an eye on their unborn child's movements and notify their healthcare practitioner of any notable changes.

Timetable for Inspections

- **Weekly Check-Ups**: To make sure the baby stays in the head-down position throughout the last few weeks of pregnancy, weekly check ups are advised.

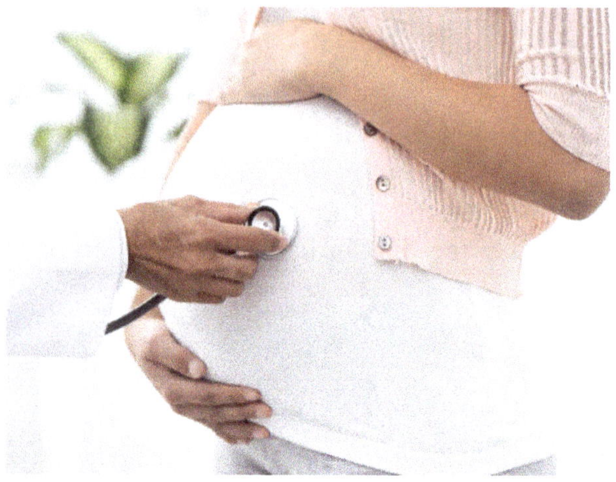

- **Bi-weekly Check-Ups**: If the pregnancy is developing well and there are no additional risk factors, bi-weekly check-ups may be adequate in some circumstances.

Role of Technology in Monitoring

- **Home Monitoring gadgets**: Parents may watch their baby's location and movements with the aid of a variety of home monitoring gadgets. Despite their potential benefits, these gadgets shouldn't take the place of routine medical examinations with doctors.

- **Telemedicine**: For routine follow-ups, parents who might find it difficult to attend in-person sessions might benefit from virtual consultations and telemedicine.

Getting Ready for Labor and Delivery

Being mentally and physically ready for labor and delivery is just one aspect of the complex process of labor preparation. Following a successful turn, parents should concentrate on last-minute details to guarantee a seamless and enjoyable birthing process.

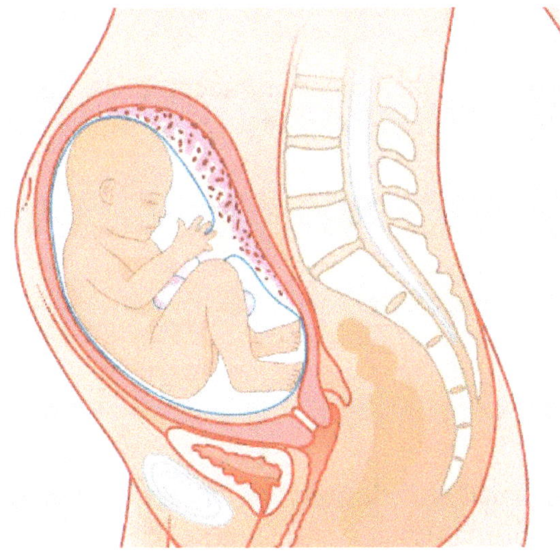

Last-minute arrangements and birth plans

- **Examining Birth Plans:** With their healthcare practitioner, parents should go over their birth plans and make any required revisions in light of the baby's current position.

- **Hospital or Birth Center Packing**: It's important to have a thoughtful hospital pack ready. This should contain any relevant paperwork and birth plans, as well as vital supplies for the mother and child.

- **Putting in Place Help Systems:** Having a birth partner, doula, or family nearby may offer a great deal of emotional and practical help throughout labor and delivery.

Physical Preparation

- **Movement and Exercise**: Consistently engaging in mild exercise can assist preserve physical preparation for childbirth. Exercises like swimming, yoga for pregnant women, and walking might be helpful.

- **Pelvic Floor activities:** During labor and delivery, strengthening the pelvic floor muscles with activities like Kegels might be beneficial.

- **Nutrition and Hydration**: Eating a well-balanced diet and drinking plenty of water is essential for a woman's general health and energy levels throughout delivery.

Psychological and Emotional Readiness

- **Childbirth Education Classes**: Learning useful skills and information for handling labor and delivery might come from taking childbirth education classes.

- **Stress-Reduction and Relaxation Techniques**: Deep breathing techniques, mindfulness, and meditation are among the practices that can help you manage stress and anxiety.

- **Visualization and Positive Affirmations:** These methods can help foster a positive outlook and lessen anxiety related to childbirth and delivery.

Talking with Your Medical Professional

- Talking About Pain Management Alternatives: Making educated decisions during labor can be aided by being aware of the pain management alternatives that are available and by sharing preferences with the healthcare professional.

- **Recognizing the indications of Labor**: To receive timely medical attention, it is essential to recognize the indications of labor and to know when to visit the hospital or birth center.

- **Emergency Plans:** Being prepared for unforeseen circumstances with a well-defined emergency plan helps ease anxiety and guarantee prompt action when necessary.

Reflecting on the Journey

An essential part of giving birth is thinking back on the experience of turning a breech baby and getting ready for labor and delivery. A sense of success, emotional closure, and insightful understanding can all be obtained from this introspection.

Telling Your Story

- **Recording Birth Stories:** Composing a birth story might help you heal and think back on the event. This might include the difficulties encountered, the techniques employed to turn the infant, and the feelings experienced during the ordeal.

- **Sharing in Support Groups**: People going through comparable struggles might get support and motivation from others who are sharing their experiences in support groups or online forums.

- **Making a Memory Book**: Pregnancy and childbirth journey images, notes, and mementos may be compiled into a treasured memory book.

Getting Knowledge and Understanding

- Reflecting on Challenges and Triumphs: Giving careful thought to the difficulties encountered and the victories attained can yield insightful knowledge and a feeling of satisfaction.

- **Finding Improvement Areas**: Thinking back on the experience can also help pinpoint areas that could be improved for the next pregnancies or for counseling other women.

- **Appreciating Support Systems**: Gratitude and a sense of connection may be fostered by acknowledging and appreciating the support networks that were in place, such as family, friends, and medical professionals.

Emotional Closure

- **Processing Emotions:** Turning a breech baby and getting ready for birth may be a very emotional experience. Emotional closure can be achieved by processing these feelings via introspection, conversation, and support.

- **Celebrating Success:** It may be a happy and gratifying experience to celebrate the baby's successful turn and the following delivery.

Sources of Additional Assistance

- **Postpartum Support Groups:** During the postpartum phase, joining a postpartum support group may offer continuing support and a feeling of community.

- **Counseling and Therapy**: Counseling and therapy can provide invaluable support and healing for parents who have had substantial stress or trauma during their journey.

- **Educational Resources**: Staying up to date on topics related to parenting, postpartum care, and baby care may help one feel confident and supported in their new position as parents.

Observing Following a Successful Turn

After a breech baby is successfully rotated to face down, it is crucial to check the baby constantly to make sure it stays in this position and to handle any possible issues as soon as they arise.

Importance of Constant Monitoring

Ensuring the baby stays head-down until birth is the major objective of continuous monitoring. This is important for several reasons:

1. **Preventing Reversion**: Even after the baby has turned, there's still a chance that it will go back to being breech, particularly if the turn happened earlier than 37 weeks. Regular observation makes it possible to identify any reversal early and take appropriate action.

2. **Early issues Detection**: Healthcare professionals can identify potential issues after the baby has turned by doing routine monitoring. This can involve problems including problems with the umbilical cord or indications of fetal discomfort.

3. **Reassurance for Parents**: Constant observation helps parents feel more at ease by keeping them informed about their baby's whereabouts and health and by easing their concerns. During the last weeks of pregnancy, having peace of mind might come from knowing that the baby is under close observation.

Methods of Monitoring

Following a successful rotation, the baby's position can be observed using several techniques:

1. **Frequent Ultrasound Scans:** The most dependable way to verify the baby's location is through ultrasound scans. Depending on the particulars of each pregnancy, these scans might be conducted at regular intervals. The baby's posture may be seen thanks to ultrasound technology, which enables medical professionals to verify that the baby is still head-down.

2. **Physical examinations:** Medical professionals may also palpate the mother's belly to determine the baby's position using physical examination techniques like Leopold's procedures. During these techniques, the baby's head, back, and buttocks are felt to ascertain its position.

3. **Fetal Movement Monitoring**: It is recommended that parents keep an eye on their unborn child's movements and notify their healthcare professional of any notable variations. A baby may have changed positions or may be experiencing a possible issue if there is a discernible reduction in movements or a change in the pattern of motions.

Schedule of Check-Ups

The particulars of the pregnancy will determine how frequently checks are needed, however as a general rule of thumb:

1. **Weekly Check-Ups**: To make sure the baby stays in the head-down position throughout the last few weeks of pregnancy, weekly check-ups are advised. Physical tests and ultrasonography scans are two possible components of these checkups.

2. **Bi-weekly Check-Ups:** If the pregnancy is developing well and there are no additional risk factors, bi-weekly check-ups may be adequate in certain circumstances. The mother and baby's unique demands will be taken into consideration by the healthcare practitioner while determining the best timetable.

Getting Ready for Delivery and Labor

Physical, mental, and emotional preparedness are all important components of the whole process of getting ready for labor and delivery. Once a breech baby has been successfully turned face down, expectant parents should concentrate on last-minute arrangements to guarantee a smooth and enjoyable birthing process.

Examining Birth Plans

Examining and completing the birth plan with the healthcare professional is one of the first stages in getting ready for labor and delivery. Preferences for labor and delivery, such as methods of pain management, labor positions, and any unique factors dependent on the baby's position, are detailed in a birth plan. It can be essential to revise the birth plan for parents who have successfully flipped a breech baby to account for the new position as well as any special needs or preferences.

Packing for a Birth Center or Hospital

Comfort and preparedness during labor and delivery may be ensured by organizing your hospital pack properly. Essentials for the mother and child should be included in the hospital bag, such as:

- **For the Mother:** Items for relaxation (music, essential oils), birth plan, insurance information, food, comfortable attire, and toiletries.

- **For the Infant:** a going-home dress, blankets, diapers, and newborn clothes.

To prevent tension at the last minute, it is best to pack the hospital bag well in advance of the due date.

Setting Up Support Systems

An effective support network may make giving delivery much more enjoyable. A birth partner, doula, family, or friends who can offer both physical and emotional support throughout labor and delivery are examples of this. It is possible to make sure that everyone is ready and focused on the mother's comfort and well-being by going over responsibilities and expectations in advance with support personnel.

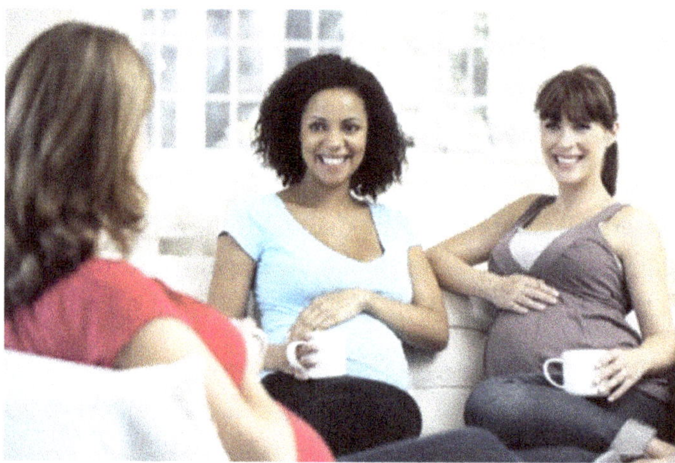

Physical Setup

Preserving one's physical health and fitness throughout pregnancy promotes general well-being and gets the body ready for delivery. Several techniques for physical preparation consist of:

- **Mild Exercise:** You may keep your strength and flexibility by doing mild activities like swimming, yoga for pregnant women, and walking.

- **Exercises for the Pelvic Floor**: Building strength in the pelvic floor muscles with exercises like Kegels can help during labor and hasten the healing process after giving birth.

- **Healthy Diet and Hydration:** Nutrition-dense, well-balanced meals, and proper hydration are essential for sustaining energy levels and meeting the demands of labor.

Psychological and Emotional Readiness

Giving birth is a life-changing event that can cause a variety of feelings. Expectant parents may face labor and delivery with confidence and resiliency by mentally and emotionally preparing:

- **Childbirth Education Classes**: Learning about the phases of labor, coping mechanisms, and medical interventions may be gained by participating in childbirth education classes. These courses equip parents to make wise choices and psychologically prepare for a range of situations.

- **Relaxation Techniques:** During labor, tension, and anxiety can be managed by using relaxation techniques such as progressive muscle relaxation, deep breathing, visualization, and meditation.

- **Positive Affirmations:** Using visualizations and affirmations that are uplifting might help people feel more empowered and ready to give birth.

Talking with Your Medical Professional

Understanding the labor and delivery process, addressing any concerns, and having an open dialogue with healthcare personnel are all dependent on open communication:

- **Talking About Pain Management Alternatives:** Parents may make well-informed decisions based on their own preferences and medical advice by being aware of the many pain relief alternatives, such as nitrous gas, epidurals, and natural pain management strategies.

- **Examining Labor Signs:** By learning the many phases and indicators of labor, parents may determine when labor starts and whether to visit a hospital or birth center.

- **Emergency Preparedness:** Working with the healthcare professional to create an emergency plan guarantees that you are ready for unforeseen circumstances during labor, such as fetal distress or issues that need immediate medical attention.

Reflecting on the Journey

It's a significant and reflective process to look back on the path of successfully turning a breech baby and getting ready for labor and delivery. Parents can obtain insights, acknowledge accomplishments, and emotionally get ready for the impending delivery experience through this introspection.

Telling Your Birth Story

Recounting the birth story and documenting it may be an effective means of capturing memories, processing feelings, and motivating those who might be going through similar difficulties. There are several ways to tell the birth story:

- **Writing**: Compose a thorough narrative of the trip that includes the breech baby's turning procedure, the feelings felt, and the exchanges with medical professionals.

- **Images and Videos**: Using images or videos to document special occasions can result in enduring memories and give the journey a visual expression.

- **Social Media or Blogs**: Posting the birth narrative on personal blogs or social media sites might help you reach a larger audience and inspire and assist others.

Thinking Back on Obstacles and Achievements

Thinking back on the difficulties and victories experienced while preparing for birth and turning a breech baby may provide insightful knowledge and foster personal development.

- **Recognizing Strengths:** Expressing gratitude for one's ability to overcome obstacles, make tough choices, and stand up for the baby's welfare.

- **Learning Opportunities:** Identifying areas for improvement or learning can help guide decisions in the future and boost self-assurance in raising children and advocating for healthcare.

- **Celebrating Milestones and Achievements:** Highlighting successes like turning a baby or facing anxieties helps people feel proud of themselves and acquire a sense of accomplishment.

Getting Over Your Emotions

Emotional closure and overall well-being are facilitated by processing feelings and experiences associated with being pregnant, giving birth, and turning a breech baby:

- **Addressing Feelings:** Emotional healing and acclimatization to motherhood are supported by expressing and processing feelings of pleasure, relief, worry, or fear related to the journey.

- **Support Systems:** During the reflective phase, talking to support systems such as a spouse, family, friends, or medical professionals may offer validation, encouragement, and reassurance.

- **Gratitude and Appreciation:** Feelings of appreciation and happiness are fostered by expressing thanks to healthcare providers, support networks, and personal assets.

Sources of Further Support

Having access to extra resources and assistance improves well-being, parental confidence, and postpartum adjustment:

- **Postpartum Support Groups:** Participating in online or local groups helps parents share knowledge, connects them with other parents going through similar experiences, and provides peer support.

- **Counseling or Therapy**: Getting help from a competent counselor or therapist offers a secure setting for processing events, exploring feelings, and creating coping mechanisms for being a parent.

- **Educational Resources:** Maintaining one's knowledge of newborn care, nursing, recuperation after childbirth, and parenting techniques builds self-assurance and encourages well-informed decision-making.

CONCLUSION

Pregnancy is a journey full of excitement, joy, and occasionally unanticipated difficulties. It can be difficult for parents to navigate the nuances of fetal positioning and delivery alternatives when their baby is breech. With the right information, encouragement, and preventative techniques, parents may actively assist their breech infant in turning over.

We have covered a wide range of topics related to breech presentation in this guide, from what it means for a baby to be breech to the advantages and disadvantages of various delivery methods. We have studied practical strategies that range from advanced medical procedures like External Cephalic Version (ECV) and holistic therapies like acupuncture and moxibustion to non-medical measures like pelvic tilts and forward-leaning inversions. To provide parents with the knowledge they need to make wise choices and actively encourage their baby to go into the ideal head-down position for delivery, each chapter has been created.

Summary of the Main Findings

1. **Comprehending Breech Presentation**: Initially, we elucidated the several varieties of breech situations and the determinants that lead to a newborn adopting this posture within the womb. Every presentation has different delivery consequences, such as the footling breech (one or both feet are positioned to enter the birth canal first) and the frank breech (buttocks first with legs folded at the hips and feet near the head).

2. **Examining Your Options:** We stressed how crucial it is to talk to healthcare experts early on about your delivery alternatives. In this conversation, the pros and cons of trying a vaginal breech delivery vs going with a scheduled cesarean section—which is frequently advised owing to safety concerns—are discussed.

3. **Non-Medical Techniques:** We gave parents thorough information on activities like pelvic tilts and forward-leaning inversions if they were interested in non-invasive techniques. By using these methods, the uterus can expand and the baby is encouraged to spontaneously turn over head-down.

4. **Medical treatments:** ECV and other medical treatments have a better success rate in flipping a baby head-down when non-medical approaches fail or when there are particular medical indications. Parents who are aware of the process, associated hazards, and necessary preparation can approach ECV with confidence.

5. **Alternative and Holistic Approaches**: To induce calm and stimulate fetal movement toward the intended position, we investigated complementary therapies such as acupuncture, moxibustion, and chiropractic adjustments (Webster technique).

6. **Problem-Solving and Troubleshooting:** We acknowledged that not all infants will turn despite attempts, and we offered advice on how to handle disappointment, and stress, and ask for more help from loved ones and medical professionals. We also spoke about situations in which professional guidance can suggest that different birth plans are necessary.

7. **Exceptional circumstances and Considerations:** We covered exceptional circumstances including multiple pregnancies and prior breech deliveries, acknowledging that every pregnancy is unique. We provided individualized counsel and extra considerations for high-risk pregnancies.

8. **Post-Turn Care and Follow-Up**: Lastly, we stressed how crucial it is to keep an eye on the baby's position following successful efforts at turning and adjust plans for labor and delivery accordingly. Being well-informed and making advance plans might help for a more seamless transition into giving birth.

Empowerment via Information and Readiness

This guide's main focus has been on empowering people via preparation and information. Parents may take an active role in their pregnancy by being aware of the mechanics of breech presentation and the resources available to encourage fetal relocation. Parents may make decisions that are in line with their preferences and the advice of their healthcare practitioner since every approach and intervention that has been described has been supported by research and is guided by pragmatic considerations.

Mental and Emotional Assistance

We understand that managing a breech presentation has an emotional and psychological impact in addition to the physical methods and medical considerations. It is normal for parents to feel a variety of emotions, such as optimism, determination, worry, and anxiety. During this period, feeling resilient and empowered can be facilitated by exploring relaxation methods like hypnobirthing, asking for help from partners and loved ones, and being open with healthcare practitioners.

Looking Forward

Remember that every step you take in preparation for your baby's birth—whether it's a scheduled cesarean section or a successful turning maneuver—is an expression of your dedication to their health. Have faith in the process, keep yourself informed, and rely on your support system for direction and inspiration. Your journey to bring your child into the world is a meaningful one, full of opportunities and very moving experiences.

Resources for Ongoing Assistance

We've included helpful appendices with resources to help you along the way, such as a dictionary of words, a list of recommended practitioners, example workout programs, and a checklist for talking with your healthcare provider about birth preparations. These tools are intended to supplement the data in this guide and act as a resource while you go through the last phases of your pregnancy and get ready for your baby's birth.